AN INTERNATIONAL PERSPECTIVE ON THE FUTURE OF RESEARCH IN CHRONIC FATIGUE SYNDROME

Edited by **Christopher R. Snell**

An International Perspective on the Future of Research in Chronic Fatigue Syndrome
Edited by Christopher R. Snell

Published by InTech
Janeza Trdine 9, 51000 Rijeka, Croatia

Publishing Process Manager Anja Filipovic

Technical Editor Teodora Smiljanic

Cover Designer InTech Design Team

Additional hard copies can be obtained from orders@intechopen.com

An International Perspective on the Future of Research in Chronic Fatigue Syndrome,
Edited by Christopher R. Snell
p. cm.
ISBN 978-953-51-0072-0

Meet the editor

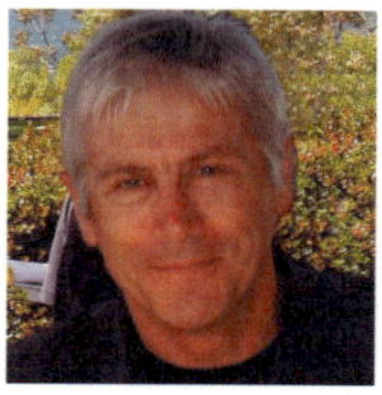

Dr Christopher Snell is a Professor of Health and Exercise Science at the University of the Pacific, Stockton, California. He is also Scientific Director of the Pacific Fatigue Laboratory, a research, clinical and teaching laboratory focused on the functional aspects of chronic fatigue syndrome/myalgic encephalomyelitis (CFS/ME) and other fatigue-related disorders. Dr Snell has been involved in CFS research for over 15 years and currently chairs the Chronic Fatigue Advisory Committee to the US Department of Health.

Contents

Preface

"It is an ill wind that blows nobody any good" would seem an apt epitaph for recent events surrounding Chronic Fatigue Syndrome (CFS) and the retrovirus XMRV. Despite the general failure to find support for a link between XMRV and CFS pathophysiology, the controversy served to shine a spotlight on CFS that may ultimately benefit the many patients around the world suffering from this poorly understood and most devastating illness. As advanced biomedical research techniques are increasingly applied to the study of CFS, it is surely only a matter of time before biomarkers are identified, etiologies understood, and remedies devised.

The goal of this book is to provide scientists, physicians, and other interested parties, access to current thinking and research findings on CFS from around the world. To this end there are five chapters originating from four different countries and three continents. They focus on topics ranging from a discussion of possible links between CFS and viral infections to the role of cardiovascular dysfunction in CFS symptoms. There are also three chapters devoted to gene research and the potential for finding a genetic origin for CFS.

Chapter 1, "Chronic Fatigue Syndrome and Viral Infections", begins with a brief history of viral research and the link between viruses and disease. It goes on to discuss the many viruses that have been implicated in CFS pathology and relevant research findings. In the absence of any definitive conclusions regarding a viral etiology for CFS, the authors hypothesize a "hit and run" effect whereby viruses trigger an illness and then disappear or that CFS is neither caused by a virus, nor an infectious disease. They do observe that should a viral cause for CFS be identified, this would greatly improve the chances of finding effective treatments for the disease.

Chapter 2, "Gene Expression in Chronic Fatigue Syndrome", presents a review of current research on gene expression and the multisystem pathophysiology of CFS. Difficulties in treating CFS are ascribed to the high-variability of genetic anomalies observed in persons with CFS. Among the most consistent findings are changes in immune-related genes. However, it is not clear whether these changes are cause or effect, highlighting the need for further study. It is recommended that future research focus on the identification of those changes in gene expression that can explain the disease profile in CFS.

Chapter 3, "Integrated Analysis of Gene Expression and Genotype Variation Data for Chronic Fatigue Syndrome", describes how by integrating genotype variation data and gene expression data, it is possible to identify potential genetic causal mechanisms in CFS. Research employing the described integrated statistical model (ISM) is presented to show how genetic pathways identified using this approach may be implicated in some CFS symptoms. The application of this integrated, two-step approach to the analysis of any heterogeneous data sets is also discussed as are potential dangers inherent to oversimplification of the causal model used for complex diseases such as CFS.

Chapter 4, "Corticosteroid-Binding Globulin Gene Mutations and Chronic Fatigue/Pain Syndromes: An Overview of Current Evidence". In addition to its role in the transport of cortisol, corticosteroid-binding globulin (CBG) may have an even broader role in the neurobehavioral response to stress. Data from both genetic epidemiological research and animal studies is presented to show links between CBG gene polymorphisms and risk for chronic fatigue and/or pain syndromes. Because this association is not universal, an interaction between phenotype and other genetic or environmental factors is proposed with further study necessary to identify the mechanisms whereby CBG may influence the stress response.

Chapter 5, "Small Heart as a Constitutive Factor Predisposing to Chronic Fatigue Syndrome", suggests a cardiac dysfunction hypothesis to explain symptoms of CFS and a common co-morbidity, orthostatic intolerance (OI). Low cardiac output due to a small left ventricular (LV) chamber, characteristic of small heart syndrome, is proposed as a contributory factor in the development of CFS. The symptoms found in persons diagnosed with small heart syndrome are shown to be very similar to those of CFS. Studies showing evidence of small heart in persons with CFS and OI are also discussed. Possible treatments aimed at improving cardiac output in this CFS subgroup are suggested along with advice on avoiding triggers that may lead to reductions in stroke volume.

While the chapters in this book are a long way from solving the enigma that is CFS, they do represent important attempts to understand this complex and perplexing disease. A common theme in them all is CFS as a multisystem disease with the possibility of more than one cause and influenced by a variety of interacting factors. They also represent what is a most welcome advance in the approach to CFS research. Theirs is a straightforward application of scientific principles and techniques toward the advancement of knowledge with the implicit recognition that this is a disease of biological origins. Further, they acknowledge the reality of CFS for persons with this disease and the importance of finding causes, treatments and ultimately a cure.

Christopher R. Snell, PhD
University of the Pacific, Stockton, CA,
USA

1

Chronic Fatigue Syndrome and Viral Infections

Frédéric Morinet[1,*] and Emmanuelle Corruble[2]
[1]*Hospital Saint-Louis,*
Center of Innovative Therapy in Oncology and Hematology (CITOH),Paris,
[2]*Paris XI University, INSERM U 669, Department of Psychiatry,*
Bicêtre University Hospital, Assistance Publique–Hôpitaux de Paris,
France

1. Introduction

The dream of all clinicians and researchers is to give their name to an illness, whatever the technique used to make the discovery. During the 20th century and the early part of the 21st century, several viruses have been identified by different procedures. Using electron microscopy, Epstein and Barr (Epstein *et al.*, 1965) detected a Herpes virus in the lymphoid cells of a native African boy with a jaw tumor identified by the surgeon, Denis Burkitt (Burkitt, 1962). A few years later, using electrosyneresis, Blumberg detected the Hepatitis B antigen in the blood of an Australian aborigine (Blumberg *et al.*, 1967, 1965). This immunological procedure was also used in 1975 by Yvonne Cossart to detect human parvovirus B19 in the serum of a blood donor in London (Cossart *et al.*, 1975).

In the last decade, molecular biology techniques have prevailed for identifying new viruses. The viruses of Hepatitis C (Choo *et al.*, 1989), Kaposi sarcoma (Chang *et al.*, 1994) and Merkel carcinoma (Feng *et al.*, 2008) have been detected in blood samples and skin biopsies. After detection, polymerase chain reaction (PCR) has been used routinely to identify pathogens. PCR is a specific and highly sensitive procedure. Its sensitivity explains the false positive results due to DNA contamination and great caution is required when positive PCR results are obtained.

There are several reasons why viral infections have long been suspected to be the cause of Chronic Fatigue Syndrome (CFS). Most patients report that their symptoms started suddenly with a flu-like illness. It is also known that some viruses, especially polio (an enterovirus), can produce a syndrome of permanent post-infection fatigue. Many people with CFS also have unusual immunological activity which might result from viral infections or predispose them to such infections. Nevertheless, at present the role of viruses in CFS remains unresolved, as it is for many autoimmune diseases such as type I diabetes and multiple sclerosis. If their precise etiological role remains elusive, despite their *in vivo* persistence, it seems that viruses may trigger the disease and then vanish. This mechanism, termed "hit and run", was described initially in bovine papillomatosis. Bovine papillomavirus is detected only at the initial stage of infection and never at the neoplastic stage (Favre, personal communication). Consequently, it may be that when a clinical diagnosis of CFS is made, it is too late to detect any possibly causative virus.

* Corresponding Author

Finally, finding a viral etiology for CFS would open the door to specific therapy that would bring hope to patients.

After presenting a summary of CFS, we shall describe viral candidates and try, with the help of examples, to explore some possible mechanisms of virus infection.

2. Background

Interest in CFS increased in the early 1980s after an epidemic of neurological symptoms, referred to as "myalgic encephalomyelitis" (ME), occurred among the staff of a London hospital. Nowadays, CFS refers to the range of complaints found in ME, or chronic fatigue and immune dysfunction syndrome (Prins *et al.*, 2006). CFS is characterized by persistent and unexplained fatigue, resulting in severe impairment of daily functioning.

2.1 Definition of CFS

The most widely supported scientific definition of CFS, which is now considered the standard, is that made in 1994 by the US Center for Disease Control and Prevention (Fukuda *et al.*, 1994). In this definition, the illness is identified by the presence of subjective symptoms, disability and absence of other explanatory illnesses, and not by objective validators, such as physical signs or abnormalities detectable by laboratory tests or imaging techniques (Prins *et al.*, 2006).

Criteria of CFS are the following:

- Persistent or relapsing unexplained chronic fatigue
- Fatigue lasting for at least 6 months
- Fatigue of new or definite onset
- Fatigue not resulting from an organic disease or from continuing exertion
- Fatigue not alleviated by rest
- Fatigue resulting in a substantial reduction in previous occupational, educational, social and personal activities
- Four or more of the following symptoms, concurrently present for 6 months: impaired memory or concentration, sore throat, tender cervical or axillary lymph nodes, muscle pain, pain in several joints, new headaches, non-refreshing sleep, or malaise after exertion

Are excluded:

- Medical condition explaining fatigue
- Major depressive disorder (psychotic features) or bipolar disorder
- Schizophrenia, dementia or delusional disorder
- Anorexia nervosa, bulimia nervosa
- Alcohol or substance abuse
- Severe obesity.

2.2 Epidemiology and clinical signs

The prevalence of CFS among adults ranges from 0.25% to 0.5%, with higher rates in women (75%) than men (25%), and more frequent in people of lower educational attainment and occupational status. The estimated prevalence is lower among children and adolescents than in adults.

CFS begins generally in young adults. The main complaint is of a persistent, severe fatigue, frequently associated with pain (mainly myalgia and headache), cognitive dysfunction, and/or gastrointestinal problems. These symptoms result in substantial reduction in occupational, educational, social, and personal activities. A thorough history, a meticulous physical and mental status examination and a range of laboratory tests and an assessment of fatigue severity and functional impairment are needed to diagnose CFS.

Initially, CFS was compared with neurasthenia (Afari *et al.*, 2003). Psychiatric comorbidities, especially depressive disorders, are commonly found (Afari *et al.*, 2003; Choa *et al.*, 2006).

Full recovery from CFS without treatment is rare. Poorer outcomes are predicted with psychiatric comorbidities and a better outcome may be predicted where there is a lower baseline fatigue (Prins *et al.*, 2006).

2.3 Etiology

The potential roles of many somatic and psychosocial factors in the etiology of CFS have been explored (Prins *et al.*, 2006), including: viral infections, immune dysfunction, neuroendocrine disorders, central nervous system dysfunction, muscle structure, exercise capacity, sleep patterns, genetics, personality, and neuropsychological processes. Both etiology and pathogenesis are probably multifactorial. To explain this complex disorder, interactions between predisposing, precipitating and perpetuating factors have been proposed.

Among predisposing factors, personality (neuroticism and introversion), lifestyle and genetics have been suggested. Among precipitating factors that might trigger the onset of CSF, acute physical stress, such as infection (flu-like illness, infectious mononucleosis, Q fever and Lyme disease), serious injuries, surgery, pregnancy, labor and psychological stress such as major life events have been cited.

3. DNA viruses

3.1 Herpes virus

The Herpes virus family includes DNA lymphotropic and neurotropic viruses. Epstein-Barr virus (EBV), Kaposi sarcoma virus (HHV-8) and cytomegalovirus (CMV) are lymphotropic whereas Herpes simplex virus (HSV), Varicella-zoster virus (VZV) and human Herpes virus 6 (HHV-6) are neurotropic. After an acute infection, these viruses persist *in vivo* and may reactivate during immunosuppression or after a stress. All, except EBV and HHV-8 are accessible to antiviral agents. For EBV and HHV- 8, reduction of immunosuppression seems to be sufficient.

3.1.1 Herpes virus and disease

There are two types of Herpes simplex virus: type 1 causes oral lesions whereas type 2 causes genital lesions. The skin lesions are typically vesicular. With the type 2 virus, the main problem is that if genital lesions occur during pregnancy, there is a risk of transmission to the neonate at delivery. With the type 1 virus, there is a risk of encephalitis, but this is very rare and depends on the patient's genetic background. Herpes simplex encephalitis is due to a series of monogenic primary immunodeficiencies that impair TLR3 and UNC-93B-dependent production of INF-alpha/beta and Interferon lambda in the central nervous system, at least in a small number of children (Sancho-Shimizu *et al.*, 2007). Consequently, it would seem that treatment of Herpes simplex encephalitis with INF-alpha, as well as with acyclovir, could improve prognosis. Encephalitis may also occur during infection by HHV-6, principally in immunocompromised patients. With lymphotropic viruses, the clinical signs are essentially seen in immunodeficient patients, such as organ transplant and bone marrow recipients and HIV patients. EBV induces lymphoma, HHV-8 is the viral agent of Kaposi sarcoma and lymphoma, and CMV is the agent of interstitial pneumonia and retinitis.

3.1.2 Herpes virus and CFS

Herpes virus is a popular hypothetical candidate for the pathogenesis of CFS, either by primary infection or after the reactivation of a latent infection. Two Herpes viruses, EBV and HHV-6, are suspected of playing a role in the development of CFS.

Prospective cohort studies have suggested that acute EBV infection triggers a post-infective syndrome in approximately 10% of patients, when evaluated 6 months after onset. Nevertheless, in a pilot study, serological patterns of anti-EBV antibody in the patients with CFS were not different from those who recovered promptly (Cameron *et al.*, 2010). In addition, the levels of circulating EBV DNA were within the range found in healthy blood donors. Finally, in a double-blind, placebo-controlled study, acyclovir therapy in patients with CFS and persistent EBV antibodies did not improve CFS (Strauss *et al.*, 1988). These findings must, however, be interpreted carefully since using acyclovir to treat EBV infection is questionable (personal data). In another study, valgancyclovir, an oral pro-drug of ganciclovir, was used to treat CFS patients with high EBV antibody titers (Kogelnik *et al.*, 2006; Lerner *et al.*, 2001). Clinical improvement was observed with a decrease in EBV antibody titer. These findings must be confirmed, but we cannot exclude the possibility that the drug has an immunomodulatory effect. Indeed, like acyclovir, valgancyclovir is not an ideal drug to treat EBV reactivation.

Because HHV-6 causes a life-long, ineradicable infection, and because of its broad tissue tropism, it has been reasonable to speculate that it might be a trigger and perpetuating factor for CFS (Komaroff, 2006). The similarities between CFS and several neurological diseases associated with HHV-6 have reinforced this speculation. In post-transplant patients, HHV-6 in the CNS causes cognitive dysfunction and fatigue similar to that reported by CFS patients. Human HHV-6 isolates are classified into two variants, termed HHV-6A (neurotropic) and HHV-6B, on the basis of their distinct genetic, antigenic and biological characteristics, but the specific pathogenicity of each variant remains poorly understood. Yalcin detected equal frequencies of HHV-6A and HHV-6B in 13 patients with CFS (Yalcin *et al.*, 1994).

Clinical studies with antiviral drugs that have *in vitro* activity against HHV-6 (for example foscarnet) could provide strong evidence for, or against, any link between HHV-6 infection and development of CFS.

3.2 Parvovirus

Autonomous parvoviruses, known to infect man, comprise parvovirus B19 and the recently discovered PARV4 and human bocavirus. PARV4 was originally detected in plasma from a patient with an "acute infection syndrome" resembling that of primary human immunodeficiency virus (HIV) infection. PARV4 is known to be widespread, specifically in people with a history of parenteral exposure (injecting drug users, hemophiliacs, polytransfused patients), with a strikingly higher incidence amongst those infected with HIV. Human bocavirus was originally found in the respiratory tracts of young children. Although it is frequently detected by PCR in the nasopharynx of viremic patients with primary lower respiratory tract infections, other co-infecting respiratory viruses are frequently detected (Servant *et al.*, 2010). As far we know, only parvovirus B19 is involved in CFS.

3.2.1 Parvovirus B19 and disease

Discovered in 1975 (Cossart *et al.*,1975), B19 can cause a wide range of mild and self-limiting clinical signs, such as *erythema infectiosum* (fifth disease) and oligoarthritis (Servant *et al.*, 2010). B19V infection may also cause acute anemia due to aplastic crisis in patients with shortened red cell survival and the chronic anemia of immunocompromised patients, i.e. HIV patients and those with congenital immunodeficiency, undergoing chemotherapy for malignancies or after organ transplant. It may also result in *hydrops fetalis* or fetal death. Erythroid progenitor cells are specifically targeted through expression of globoside P antigen, which acts as the receptor for B19 virus, explaining the development of anemia. Recently, cases of neurological signs and myocardial infections have been associated with B19 infection and the spectrum of B19-linked diseases may increase further. The primary route of B19V transmission is the respiratory tract (via aerosols), with a majority of infections occurring during childhood. The infection may also be transmitted by organ transplant and especially by transfusion of blood components, in particular packed red cells from blood collected during the short pre-seroconversion viremic phase. In classical natural history, an acute B19V infection occurring in immunologically competent individuals is controlled by neutralizing antibodies. A transient, high level viremia lasts for less than one week and declines with the appearance of specific IgM antibodies, which persist for eight to ten weeks, followed by the appearance of life-long specific IgG antibodies. Persistent infection may be observed in immunocompromised patients unable to produce neutralizing antibodies able to clear the virus, leading to chronic B19V carriage with or without anemia. In this case, an infusion of immunoglobulins is necessary. However, even if the immune response of healthy subjects is able to clear infection and provide life-long protection against B19V, persistence of infection has been reported in the bone marrow of immunocompetent subjects with or without symptoms, and recently persisting low levels of B19V DNA were found in the blood of some immunocompetent subjects several years after primary infection. The mechanism of such chronic B19V carriage remains unclear.

3.2.2 Parvovirus B19 and CFS

McGhee (McGhee *et al.*, 2005) reported the case of a 16-year-old boy with no evidence of immunodeficiency who had a 2-year history of chronic fatigue, low-grade fever and slapped-cheek rash associated with a chronic parvovirus B19 viremia that was detected by quantitative PCR. Parvovirus B19 titers for IgG and IgM were strongly positive. Three months of high dose (total 560 g) intravenous immunoglobulin (IVIG) was required before both symptoms and viremia resolved. Slapped-check rash is not included in the diagnostic criteria of CFS, so in this case we must speak of chronic fatigue rather than CFS. It is not known whether his improvement and that of other patients described in the literature by Kerr *et al.* results from increased titers of specific antibody or is due to the immunomodulatory effects of high dose IVIG (Kerr *et al.*, 2003). Whatever the mechanism, it seems that IVIG is a promising treatment for the chronic fatigue following Parvovirus B19 infection. Kerr (Denavur & Kerr, 2006) claimed that acute symptomatic parvovirus B19 infection is associated with elevated circulating TNF-alpha and IFN-gamma and may be followed by CFS. Nevertheless Barbara Cameron, by analyzing serum cytokine levels in post-infective fatigue syndrome patients and in healthy controls, found no statistically significant differences in serum levels of any cytokines at any time (Cameron *et al.*, 2010).

3.3 Other DNA viruses

Two other DNA viruses have been unsuccessfully associated to CFS. Firstly, the human polyomavirus JC which causes progressive multifocal leukoencephalopathy, and which infects granule cell neurons in the cerebellum and sometimes infects grey matter. It may also cause meningitis (Tan & Koralnik, 2010). JC virus-induced disorders are essentially observed in immunosuppressed patients, whether or not HIV positive. There is no specific antiviral drug against the JC virus and the goal of current treatment is to restore the host's adaptive immune response to the JC virus so as to control infection. At present, there is no proof that JC virus induces CFS. The second virus putatively associated with CFS is a circovirus, the TTvirus. Circoviruses have a questionable pathogenicity in man, but in animals they may infect the brain and cause disease, e.g., post-weaning multisystemic wasting syndrome of pigs (Hino, 2002). Only one report suggests that TTvirus may induce CFS (Grinde, 2008). Further studies are necessary to implicate TTvirus, a non-pathogenic virus, in this syndrome.

4. RNA viruses

4.1 Enterovirus

Infection by enterovirus in man, although often asymptomatic, is responsible for a wide range of acute diseases (Morinet, 2008). In addition, they are possibly involved in the genesis of chronic enterovirus diseases, including chronic myocardial diseases, post-poliomyelitis syndrome and even juvenile-onset (type1) diabetes mellitus (see below). The role of enteroviruses in the pathogenesis of CFS, an old saga, has been largely disputed The detection, over a long period of time, of enterovirus structural proteins (VP-1 in sera) and enterovirus RNA in the muscle biopsy specimens of patients with CFS is disturbing (Douche-Aourik, 2003). Gow (Gow *et al.*, 1994) investigated a large number of muscle biopsies from patients with either CFS or neuromuscular disorders and demonstrated the presence of enteroviral RNA by RT-PCR in 26.4% and 19.8% of samples respectively. It is necessary to demonstrate enterovirus within the muscle fibres by *in situ* PCR to prove that viral persistence alters the metabolism of the cells and thus show that such abnormalities cause clinical symptoms (Dalakas, 2003).

4.2 Other RNA viruses

A case report recently described an adolescent boy who was diagnosed as suffering from CFS five months after infection with H1N1 influenza (Vallings, 2010). Laboratory test results were normal. Other articles investigated the role of GB virus in CFS (Jones *et al.*, 2005; Sullivan *et al.*, 2011). GB virus, a flavivirus, has many properties that require study to assess its possible association with CFS; effectively this virus replicates preferentially in peripheral blood mononuclear cells, primarily B and T lymphocytes, and in bone marrow *in vivo*. Nevertheless, two of twelve CFS patients and one of 21 healthy controls were seropositive for GB virus; consequently there is no evidence this virus is associated with CFS.

Among RNA viruses, there have been conflicting findings with the neurotropic, negative-stranded RNA Borna virus (De la Torre, 2002). This virus is the causative agent of Borna disease, a sporadic and often fatal neurological disease of horses and sheep in central Europe and which has been known since the 18th century (Schwemmle, 2001). The mode of transmission is unknown but is thought to be by saliva, or nasal and conjunctival secretions. Serological and molecular epidemiological studies suggest that such a virus can infect man (Nowotny & Kolodziejek, 2000). Despite enormous efforts from many laboratories, it is still unclear whether Borna virus infection is associated with human psychiatric disease and CFS. Inadvertent sample contamination has been suggested (Durrwald *et al.*, 2007; Schwemmle 2001; Evengard *et al.*, 1999).

Finally, two studies have reported that most CFS patients harbour a gamma retrovirus, the xenotropic murine leukemia-related virus (XMRV) in blood (Kearney & Maldarelli, 2010; Lombardi *et al.*, 2009). This finding has raised speculation that it may cause the syndrome. However, four other laboratories could not replicate this finding, whilst four new studies found it only as a laboratory contaminant (Calaway, 2011; Cohen, 2011; Kaiser, 2011; Schutzer *et al.*, 2011; Shin *et al.*, 2011; Kean, 2010; Mayor, 2010; Sato *et al.*, 2010; Stoye *et al.*,2010; Coffin & Stoye, 2009). In 2011, at a retrovirology meeting in Boston, Massachusetts, researchers presented evidence that this retrovirus is, in effect, a laboratory artefact and not a human pathogen.

5. Viral persistence

A virus must have two essential characteristics in order to persist in a host (De la Torre *et al.*, 1991). Firstly, the virus, by any one of several means, must escape the host's immunological surveillance. One classical mechanism is virus-induced down-regulation of HLA class I. The infected cell becomes invisible to TCD8+ cytotoxic lymphocytes. This mechanism is used extensively by Herpes viruses. The Herpes virus group is unique in that virtually all people have latent infections in their peripheral ganglia and/or their white blood cells, which may be reactivated to cause symptomatic disease, even decades after initial infection. One such virus, the Varicella Zoster Virus, induces shingles (zoster) many years after varicella infection in infancy. Virtually all the symptoms of shingles occur also in CFS, except for the painful rash (Shapiro, 2009). Secondly, the virus must generate defective particles and variants that diminish the expression of its gene product. For example the measles virus, after a primary infection, causes systemic disease with a typical skin rash. But during its replication it produces defective particles which persist in the CNS where their accumulation may lead to subacute sclerosing panencephalitis after ten years. This disease is prevented by measles vaccination.

Another mechanism by which persistent virus infection produced disease was uncovered after the discovery that some viruses could alter cell differentiation (i.e. the "luxury" function of cells), without causing cell destruction, and thereby altering homeostasis. For example, whilst examining the effects of persistent lymphocytic choriomeningitis virus (an RNA virus which infects mice) infection on differentiated neuroblastoma cells, Oldstone (Oldstone *et al.*, 1982) noted abnormalities in the synthesis and degradation of the neurotransmitter acetylcholine caused by decreased production of the appropriate acetylase or esterase enzyme. Nevertheless, these neuroblastoma cells were of normal morphology, growth rate, cloning efficiency and in levels of total RNA, DNA, protein and vital enzyme synthesis. Infected cells were indistinguishable from infected ones by both light and high resolution electromicroscopy. In man, after infection with influenza virus, peripheral blood lymphocytes no longer performed their expected specialized functions, including antibody synthesis and they no longer had the capacity to act as killer cells (Oldstone, 2002). Hence, this human RNA virus altered the different cell functions without lysing or destroying them. Viruses act very subtly on a cell and disorder its function, but not so severely as to kill the infected cell. Yet, for the host, the end result is perturbed homeostasis and disease.

Persistent enterovirus infections have been implicated in a number of chronic human diseases including dilated cardiomyopathy, chronic muscle disorders, type I diabetes mellitus and myalgia encephalomyelitis/CFS. Chia (Chia *et al.*, 2010) demonstrated the presence of enterovirus protein, viral RNA and the replication of non-cytopathic viruses from stomach biopsies from CFS patients, years after the initial acute flu-like illness. More interestingly, in a prospective, longitudinal study of three patients, all developed acute enterovirus infections, documented by the presence of enteroviral RNA in the secretions, blood or affected tissues, and, over the next few years, this was followed by a range of symptoms consistent with CFS. Years after acute infections with respiratory/gastrointestinal symptoms, viral protein and RNA were found in stomach biopsies. Chronic infections in immunocompetent hosts may represent stalemate between attenuated, intracellular viruses and an ineffective immune response.

6. Hit and run

Over the past twenty years, no study has found conclusive evidence of an infectious etiological agent for CFS. The disorder is complex and multifactorial; nevertheless we cannot exclude the possibility that some infectious agent may trigger the disorder and then vanish. This mechanism, termed "hit and run" is well known in virology. *In vitro*, B cell cancers tend to maintain gammaherpesvirus genomes, whereas Kaposi's sarcoma and nasopharyngeal carcinoma tend to lose them (Stevenson *et al.*, 2010). In bovine papillomatosis, at the stage of *in situ* carcinoma, viral sequences are no longer detected. It also seems that the HTLV-1 Tax protein is absent at the final step of leukemia/lymphoma. Outside the field of oncology, paramyxovirus and respiratory viruses exhibit a "hit and run" phenomenon indicated by the development of asthmatic symptoms long after the infection has cleared (Holtzman *et al.*, 2004). A single paramyxoviral infection of mice (C57BL6/J strain) not only produces acute bronchiolitis but also triggers a chronic response with airway hyper-reactivity and goblet cell hyperplasia lasting for at least a year after complete viral clearance (Walter *et al.*, 2002). A "hit and run" event may also occur where antibodies to a virus recognize similar amino-acid sequences or patterns found in host cells. This cross-reactivity is termed molecular mimicry and does not require a replicating agent, and an immune mediated injury may occur after the immunogen has been removed (Oldstone, 1998).

7. Conclusion

CFS is a common problem and all clues as to its possible cause are welcome. Despite intense efforts, no virus has been clearly incriminated. Their detection seems more casual that causal. In addition, the study of viral infections in monozygotic twins who are discordant for CFS does not suggest that a virus is the culprit (Koelle *et al.*, 2002). The recent association of XMRV with CFS re-opens the debate about laboratory contamination; whether the detection of this gammaretrovirus indicates a real infection or whether it is due to a laboratory artefact remains highly controversial. If the findings linking XMRV with CFS are not due to laboratory artefacts, how can we explain the failure of other investigators to replicate the findings? Different inclusion criteria for CFS cannot account for the difference between 0% and 67% found in the laboratories (Weiss, 2010).

One over-arching question is the following: is CFS an infectious disease? If this is the case, despite the absence of supporting data, patients with CFS must abstain from blood donation, as has been suggested by Bridget M. Kuehn (Kuehn, 2010) in a provocative editorial of the JAMA. At present, there has been no confirmation that transfusion is associated with the disease.

8. References

Afari N.&Buchwald D (2003).Chronic Fatigue Syndrome: A Review. *Am J Psychiatry*, Vol. 160, 221–236.

Blumberg BS., Gerstley BJ., Hungerford DA., London WT. & Sutnick AI.(1967) A serum antigen (Australia antigen) in Down's syndrome, leukemia and hepatitis. *Ann Intern Med*, Vol. 66, 924-931

Blumberg BS., Alter HJ. & Vinisch SA.(1965) A "new antigen in leukemia sera. *JAMA*, Vol. 191, 541-546

Burkitt D. (1962) A children's cancer dependent on climatic factors. *Nature*, Vol. 194, 232-234

Callaway E. (2011) Fighting For A Cause. *Nature*, Vol. 471, 282-285

Cameron B., Flamand L., Juwana H., Middeldorp J., Naing Z., Rawlinson W., Ablashi D. & Lloyd A. (2010) Serological and Virological Investigation of the Role of the Herpesviruses EBV, CMV and HHV-6 in Post-Infective Fatigue Syndrome., J Med Virol., Vol. 82, 1684-1688

Cameron B., Hirschberg DL., Rosenberg-Hassan Y., Ablashi D. & Lloyd A. (2010) Serum Cytokine Levels in Postinfective Fatigue Syndrome. *CID*, Vol. 50,

Chang Y., Cesarman E., Pessin MS., Lee F., Culpepper J., Knowles DM. & Moore P. (1994) Identification of Herpesvirus-Like DNA Sequences in AIDS-Associated Kaposi' Sarcoma. *Science*, Vol. 266,1865-1869

Chia J., Chia A., Voeller M., Lee T. & Chang R. (2010) Acute enterovirus infection followed by myalgic encephalomyelitis/chronic fatigue syndrome(ME/CFS) and viral persistence. *J.Clin.Pathol.*, Vol. 63, 165-168

Choa HJ., Skowerab A., Clearea A. & Wesselya S. (2006). Chronic fatigue syndrome: an update focusing on phenomenology and pathophysiology. *Curr Opin Psychiatry*, Vol. 19,67–73.

Choo QL., Kuo G., Weiner AJ., Overby LR., Bradley DW. & Houghton M.(1989) Isolation of a cDNA Clone Derived from a Blood-Borne Non-A, Non-B Viral Hepatitis Genome. *Science*, Vol. 244, 360-362

Coffin JM. & Stoye J. (2009) A New Virus for Old Diseases. *Science*, Vol. 326, 530-531, ISSN 0036-8075

Cohen J. (2011) More Negative Data for Link Between Mouse Virus and Human Disease. *Science*, Vol. 331, 1253-1254,ISSN 0036-8075

Cossart YE., Field AM., Cant B. & Widdows D.(1975), Parvovirus-like particles in human sera. *Lancet*, Vol. 1 (7898), 72-73

Dalakas MC. (2003) Enteroviruses in chronic fatigue syndrome: "now you see them, now you don't". *J.Neurol Neurosurg Psychiatry*, Vol. 74,1361-1362

De La Torre (2002) Bornavirus and the Brain. *JID*, Vol. 186, S241-S247

De La Torre JC., Borrow P. & Oldstone MBA.(1991) Viral persistence and disease: Cytopathology in the absence of cytolysis. *British Medical Bulletin*, Vol. 47, 838-851

Denavur LD. & Kerr JR. (2006) Chronic fatigue syndrome. *J Clin Virol.*, Vol. 37, 139-150

Douche-Aourik F., Berlier W., Féasson L., Bourlet T., Harrath R., Omar S., Grattard F., Denis C. & Pozzetto B. (2003) Detection of Enterovirus in Human Skeletal Muscle From Patients With Chronic Inflammatory Muscle Disease or fibromyalgia and Healthy Subjects. *J.Med.Virol.*, Vol. 71, 540-547

Durrwald R., Kolodziejek J., Herzog S. & Nowotny N. (2007) Meta-analysis of putative human bornavirus sequences fails to provide evidence implicating Borna disease virus in mental illness. *Rev.Med.Virol.*, Vol.17, 181-203

Epstein MA., Henle G., Achong BG & Barr YM. (1965) Morphological and biological studies on a virus in culture lymphoblasts from Burkitt's lymphoma. J Exp Med, Vol. 121, 761-770

Evengard B., Briese T., Lindh G., Lee S. & Lipkin WI. (1999)Absence of evidence of borna disease virus infection in Swedish patients with Chronic Fatigue Syndrome. *J. NeuroVirol*, Vol. 5, 495-499

Feng h., Shuda M., Chang Y. & Moore P. (2008) Clonal Integration of a Polyomavirus in Human Merkel Cell Carcinoma. *Science*, Vol. 319,1096-1100

Fukuda K., Straus SE., Hickie I., Sharpe MC., Dobbins JG., Komaroff A. & the International Chronic Fatigue Syndrome Study Group. The Chronic Fatigue Syndrome: A Comprehensive Approach to Its Definition and Study (1994). *Ann Intern Med*, Vol. 121, 953-959.

Gow JW., Behan WM., Simpson K., Mc Garry F., Keir S. & Behan PO. (1994) Studies on enterovirus in patients with chronic fatigue. *CID*, Vol.18, S126-129.

Grinde B. (2008) Is chronic fatigue syndrome caused by a rare brain infection of a common, normally benign virus? *Medical Hypotheses*, Vol. 71, 270-274

Hino S. (2002) TTV, a new human virus with single stranded circular DNA genome. *Rev Med. Virol*, Vol. 12,151-158

Holtzman MJ., Shornick LP., Grayson MH., KimEY., Tyner JW., Patel AC., Agapov E. & Zhang Y. (2004) « Hit-and-Run » effects of Paramyxoviruses as a basis for Chronic Respiratory Disease. *Pediatr Infect Dis J*, Vol. 23, S235-S245, ISSN 0891-3668/04/2311-0235

Jones JF., Kulkarni PS., Butera ST, & Reeves W. (2005) GB-virus-C- a virus without a disease: We cannot give it chronic fatigue syndrome. *BMC Infectious Diseases*, Vol. 5, 78

Kaiser, J. (2011) Studies Point to Possible Contamination in XMRV Findings. *Science*, Vol. 331, 17, ISSN 0036-8075

Kean S. (2010) An Indefatigable Debate Over Chronic Fatigue Syndrome. *Science*, Vol. 327, 254-255, ISSN 0036-8075

Kearney M. & Maldarelli F. (2010) Current Status of Xenotropic Murine Leukemia Virus-Related Retrovirus in Chronic Fatigue Syndrome and Prostate Cancer: Reach for a Scorecard, Not a Prescription Pad. *JID*, Vol. 202, 1463-1466

Kerr JR., Cunniffe VS., Kelleher P., Bernstein RM., & Bruce IN. (2003) Successful Intravenous Immunoglobulin Therapy in 3 Cases of Parvovirus B19-Associated Chronic Fatigue Syndrome. *CID*, Vol. 36,e100-6

Koelle DM., Barcy S., Huang ML., Ashley RL., Corey L., Zeh J., Ashton S & Buchwald D. (2002) Markers of viral infection in monozygotic twins discordant for chronic fatigue syndrome. *CID*, 35, 518-525

Kogelnik AQM., Loomis K., Hoegh-Petersen M., Rosso F., Hischier C. & Montoya JG. (2006) Use of valganciclovir in patients with elevated antibody titers against Human Herpesvirus6 (HHV-6) and Epstein-Barr Virus (EBV) who were experiencing central nervous system dysfunction including long-standing fatigue. *J Clin Virol*,Vol. 37, S33-S38

Komaroff AL. (2006) Is human herpesvirus-6 a trigger for chronic fatigue syndrome? *J Clin Virol.*, Vol. 37, S39-S46

Kuehn BM. (2010) Study reignites debate about viral agent in patients with chronic fatigue syndrome. *JAMA*, Vol. 304,1653-1656

Lerner AM., Zervos M., Chang CH., Beqaj S., Goldstein J., O'Neill W., Dworkin H., Fitgerald T. & Deeter RG. (2001) A Small, Randomized, Placebo-Controlled Trial of the Use of Antiviral Therapy for Patients with Chronic Fatigue Syndrome. *CID*, Vol. 32, 1657-1658

Lombardi VC., Ruscetti FW., Das Gupta J., Pfost MA., Hagen K., Peterson DL., Ruscetti SK., Bagni R.K., Petrow-Sadowski C., Gold B., Dean M., Silverman RH.& Mikovits JA. (2009) Detection of an Infectious Retrovirus, XMRV, in Blood Cells of Patients With Chronic Fatigue Syndrome. *Science*, Vol. 326, 585-589, ISSN 0036-8075

Mayor S. (2010) Study fails to show link previously found between virus chronic fatigue syndrome. *BMJ*, Vol. 340, c1033

McGhee SA., Kaska B., Liebhaber M. & Stiehm ER. (2005) Persistent Parvovirus-Associated Chronic Fatigue Treated with High Dose Intravenous Immunoglobulin. *Pediatr Infect Dis J*, Vol. 24, 3, 272-274

Morinet, F. (2008). Virus et muscles. *Revue du Rhumatisme*, Vol. 75, 169-171, ISSN 1169-8330

Nowotny N. & Kolodziejek J. (2000) Demonstration of Borna Disease Virus Nucleic Acid in a patient with Chronic Fatigue Syndrome. *JID*, Vol. 181, 1860-1861

Oldstone,MBA.(2002) Travels along the viral-immunobiology highway., *Immunologial Reviews*, Vol. 185, 54-68

Oldstone, MBA. (1998). Molecular mimicry and immune-mediated diseases. *FASEB J.*, Vol. 12, 1255-1265

Oldstone, MBA., Sinha Y.N., Blount P., Tishon A., Rodriguez M., Von Wedel R. & Lampert PW. (1982) Virus-induced alterations in Homeostasis: Alterations in differentiated Functions of Infected Cells in vivo. *Science*, Vol. 218, 1125-1127

Prins JB., van der Meer JWM. & Bleijenberg G. (2006). Chronic fatigue syndrome. *Lancet*, Vol. 367, 346–355

Sancho-Shimizu V., Zhang SY., Abel L., Tardieu M., Rozenberg F., Jouanguy E. & Casanova JL. (2007) Genetic susceptibility to herpes simplex virus 1 encephalitis in mice and humans. *Curr Opin Allergy Clin Immunol*, Vol. 7, 495-505

Sato E., Furuta RA. & Miyazawa T. (2010) An Endogenous Murine Leukemia Viral genome Contaminant in a Commercial RT-PCR Kit is Amplified Using Standard Primers for XMRV. *Retrovirology*, Vol. 7, 110

Shapiro JS., (2009) Does varicella-zoster virus infection of the peripheral ganglia cause Chronic Fatigue Syndrome?, *Medical Hypotheses*, Vol. 73, 728-734

Schutzer S., Rounds MA., Natelson BH, Ecker DJ; & Eshoo MW. (2011) Analysis of Cerebrospinal Fluid from Chronic Fatigue Syndrome Patients for Multiple Human Ubiquitous Viruses and Xenotropic Murine Leukemia-Related Virus. *Ann Neurol*,1-4

Schwemmle M.(2001) Borna disease virus infection in psychiatric patients: are we on the right track? *Lancet Infectious Diseases*, Vol. 1, 46-52

Servant-Delmas A., Lefrere JJ., Morinet F.& Pillet S. (2010) Advances in Human B19 Erythrovirus Biology. *J.Virol.*, Vol. 84, 19, 9658-9665

Shin CH., Bateman L., Schlaberg R., Bunker AM., Leonard CJ., Hughen RW., Light AR., Light KC. & Singh IR. (2011) Absence of XMRV Retrovirus and Other Murine Leukemia Virus-Related Viruses in Patients with Chronic Fatigue Syndrome. *J.Virol*, Vol. 85, 14, 7195-7202

Stevenson PG., May JS., Connor V. & Efstathiou S. (2010) Vaccination against a hit-and-run viral cancer. *J.Gen.Virol.*,Vol. 91, 2176-2185

Stoye JP., Silverman RH., Boucher CA. & Le Grice SFJ. (2010) The xenotropic murine leukemia virus-related retrovirus debate continues at first international workshop. *Retrovirology*,Vol. 7, 113

Straus S., Dale JK., Tobi M., Lawley T., Preble O., Blaese RM., Hallahan C. & Henle W. (1988) Acyclovir Treatment of the Chronic Fatigue Syndrome. *N Engl J Med*, Vol. 319, 1692-1698.

Sullivan PF., Allander T., Lysholm F., Goh S., Persson B., Jacks A., Evengard B., Pedersen NL. & Andersson B. (2011) An unbiased metagenomic search for infectious agents using monozygotic twins discordant for chronic fatigue. *BMC Microbiology*, 11,2

Tan CS. & Koralnik IJ. (2010) Progressive multifocal leukoencephalopathy and other disorders caused by JC virus: clinical features and pathogenesis. *Lancet Neurol*, Vol. 9, 425-437

Vallings R. (2010) A case of chronic fatigue syndrome triggered by influenza H1N1 (swine influenza). *J.Clin.Pathol.*, Vol. 63, 184-185

Walter, MJ., Morton JD., Kajiwara N., Agapov E. & Holtzman MJ. (2002) Viral induction of a chronic asthma phenotype and genetic segregation from the acute response. *J.Clin.invest.*, Vol. 110, 165-175

Weiss RA.(2010) A cautionary tale of virus and disease. *BMC Biology*, 8, 124

Yalcin S., Kuratsune H., Yamaguchi K., Kitani T. & Yamanishi K. (1994) Prevalence of human herpesvirus 6 variants A and B in patients with chronic fatigue syndrome *Microbiol Immunol.*, Vol. 38, 7, 587-590

2

Gene Expression in Chronic Fatigue Syndrome

Ekua W. Brenu[1,2], Kevin J. Ashton[2], Gunn M. Atkinson[2],
Donald R. Staines[1,3] and Sonya Marshall-Gradisnik[1,2]
*[1]Faculty of Health Science and Medicine,
Population Health and Neuroimmunology Unit, Bond University, Queensland,
[2]Faculty of Health Science and Medicine, Bond University, Queensland,
[3]Gold Coast Public Health Unit,
Queensland Health Robina,
Australia*

1. Introduction

Chronic Fatigue Syndrome (CFS) is a disorder of unknown origin likely affecting multiple physiological processes. CFS is often a diagnosis of exclusion following a history of 6 months or more where patients may experience partial to full recovery, relapse or a worsening in symptoms and hence deterioration in health (Brkic et al., 2011). The clinical manifestations include moderate to severe fatigue, muscle pain, swollen lymph nodes, headaches, impaired sleep and cognition (Fukuda et al., 1994). A diagnosis of CFS is made using questionnaires which include Centre for Disease Prevention and control criteria for CFS, the Australian, British and Canadian CFS classifications and the recently developed World Health Organisation's International Classification of Diseases for CFS (Carruthers et al., 2011, Carruthers et al., 2003; Fukuda et al., 1994; Lloyd et al., 1990; Sharpe et al., 1991). CFS is a heterogeneous and multifactorial disorder. Mechanisms to explain the underlying factors and processes that are responsible for disease progression and symptom profile of this disorder remains to be established. However, research has demonstrated that CFS impacts the endocrine, neurological, immune and metabolic processes resulting in impaired physiological homeostasis (Brenu et al., 2010; Demitrack, 1997; Schwartz et al., 1994). While these processes are likely compromised and collectively contribute to ill health in CFS patients, CFS remains a disorder lacking a clear molecular or biochemical cause.

Twin studies have revealed that there is no single genetic factor associated with CFS (Evengard et al., 2005). Several molecular studies have identified genes that are differentially expressed in CFS patients in comparison to non-CFS individuals (Kaushik et al., 2005, Kerr et al., 2008; Gow et al., 2009; Light et al., 2009; Saiki et al., 2008). Additionally, these expressional differences in CFS may be as a result of the multifactorial nature of CFS. The challenge is to understand the relationship between these genetic discrepancies in CFS eventuating discovery of its pathomechanism leading to appropriate treatment and ultimately a cure. Gene expression studies in CFS have shown possible links between CFS and a number of molecular pathways associated with immune, neurological and metabolic processes (Kerr et al., 2008). The purpose of this chapter is to review the literature focusing on gene expression changes and their role in the pathophysiology of CFS.

2. Molecular studies

2.1 Candidate gene studies

Candidate gene studies are mainly employed to address the biological characteristics of known genes that predispose them to have an involvement in CFS. The advantage of this approach is that it allows for the detection of common alleles with some effect on the disease presentation. Comparisons between CFS patients and non-fatigue controls on measures of allele and genotype frequencies of identified markers have shown significant differences between these groups. This method has been used to investigate the human leukocyte antigens (HLA) markers and killer cell immunoglobulin-like markers of NK receptors in CFS patients. In some CFS patients significant increases in HLA alleles, HLA-DQA1*01 and HLA-DQB1*06 have been observed compared to control participants (Smith et al. 2005). Among the killer cell immunoglobulin-like receptors (KIRs), high levels of KIR3DS1 with loss of HLA-Bw4lle80 ligands is common among CFS patients compared to control participants (Pasi et al., 2011). Similarly, other HLA haplotypes such as HLA-DRB1*1301 are elevated in CFS patients (Carlo-Stella et al., 2009). Polymorphisms in other receptors also occurs in CFS, importantly a number of the alleles for the receptor for advanced glycation end product (RAGE) may be decreased in CFS patients (Carlo-Stella et al., 2009). These changes in allelic frequencies and haplotypes especially in the HLA molecules may be associated with the inflammatory state of CFS patients.

Gene studies with SNPs may be an alternative pathway for determining susceptibility to CFS. CFS patients are more likely to have SNP variations for the glucocorticoid receptor gene *NR3C1* with high incidence of risk conferring haplotypes (Rajeevan et al., 2007). The serotonergic system in some CFS patients is compromised and this is typified by an over active 5-hydroxytryptamine (5-HT) and a down regulated hypothalamic-pituitary-adrenal (HPA) axis (Demitrack, 1997). This likely occurs as a consequence of polymorphisms in genes that regulate serotonergic signalling. Hence, in CFS an increase in the polymorphism of the A allele linked with -1438G/A in the *HTR2A* receptor may explain these compromises (Smith et al., 2008). In particular, -1438G/A has been associated with suicide and cognitive impairment (Arango et al., 2003; Reynolds et al., 2006).

2.2 Twin studies

CFS may be prevalent in some families, thus, CFS may have a heritable component. However, the credibility of this observation remains to be determined. Self report measures and restriction fragment length polymorphism are most often used to assess the hereditability of CFS (Crawley & Smith 2007). CFS may have a familial predisposition as relatives of patients with CFS may not necessarily meet the criteria for CFS but may be more prone to experience some of the symptoms of CFS (Walsh et al., 2001). Although twin studies allude to the existence of a genetic predisposition to CFS, this may be higher among monozygotic twins compared to dizygotic twins (Buchwald et al., 2001). Twins with CFS may share similar symptoms and experience the same level of severity in CFS related symptoms (Claypoole et al., 2007). Despite these heritable predispositions observed in twin studies, they are not enough to confirm a genetic basis for CFS (Albright et al., 2011).

2.3 Gene expression microarray studies

Genome wide studies using microarrays is a predictive method of determining genes that may influence unexplained disorders such as CFS for which an aetiological mechanism is lacking. These large scale explorative studies are more often extensive and are able to determine the expression levels of genes expressed in CFS and non-CFS participants. While the results from these studies may be useful, validation through real-time quantitative polymerase chain reaction is most often required to ensure that the identified genes are representative of either a down or an up-regulation in gene expression patterns. Most of these large scale studies have identified genes that are differentially expressed in CFS compared to non-fatigued participants (Cameron et al., 2007; Carmel et al., 2006; Fang et al., 2006; Kaushik et al., 2005; Kerr et al., 2008; Saiki et al., 2008; Whistler et al., 2005; Whistler et al., 2003). In general, these genes regulate important physiological activities that are compromised in CFS. These include immune, endocrine, neurologic, metabolic and cellular activities. Elucidation of genes that predispose an individual to CFS is essential in understanding the mechanism of CFS. Gene expression studies have allowed for the identification of a number of genes involved in different aspects of the disease.

2.4 CFS gene expression studies

Many factors can influence susceptibility to CFS. Changes in the expression of genes important for various physiological processes may affect normal function. The vast majority of research in CFS has confirmed significant compromise to immune, endocrine, neurological and metabolic processes. Immunological abnormalities observed in CFS patients include decreases in cytotoxic activity of Natural Killer (NK) cells and perturbations in cytokine levels.

2.4.1 Cytokine and chemokine genes

Cytokines and their genes are vital for sustaining and regulating innate and adaptive immune activities such as cell differentiation, proliferation and activation. *IL-8* is a pro-inflammatory chemokine gene with chemotactic properties for neutrophils during pathogen invasion and other immunological insults (Huber et al., 1991). In CFS *IL-8* has been shown to be significantly increased in expression in comparison to non-CFS individuals (Vernon et al., 2002). During neutrophil pathogen lysis, phagocytic products are released which acts as a positive feedback process to activate IL-8 to recruit more neutrophils (Ito et al., 2004; Sparkman and Boggaram, 2004). Alterations in *IL-8* mRNA expression is linked with inflammation (Mukaida, 2003; Nozell et al., 2006; Xie, 2001). An increase in *IL-8* expression noted in CFS patients may occur as a result of an increase in oxidative stress during inflammation (Shono et al., 1996; Ito et al., 2004; Sparkman and Boggaram, 2004). The promoter region of *IL-8* is bound and activated by transcription factors including NF-κB A substantial decrease in the expression of *NF-κB* negatively affects *IL-8* (Huang et al., 2001). *NF-κB* is a necessary component in the activation and signalling pathway of other leukocyte cytokines and reductions in their expression increases vulnerability to infectious agents and inflammatory reactions (Artis et al., 2003; Bohuslav et al., 1998; Sha et al., 1995; Campbell et al., 2000; Yang et al., 1998).

During inflammation, immune cells such as macrophages produce pro-inflammatory molecules such as TNF-α. The severity of the inflammatory response determines the level of TNF-α produced. The *TNFA* gene is contained within the MHC complex; once it has been translated it functions by binding to TNF receptors TNFR1 or TNFR2. TNF-α has a higher affinity for the TNFR2 receptor compared to the TNFR1 (Orlinick and Chao, 1998). TNFR2 modulates the proliferation of T lymphocytes and encourages pro-inflammatory responses. Usually a low concentration of TNF-α is required to activate TNFR2 while TNFR1 is stimulated in the presence of increased concentration of TNF-α. These interactions are vital for cell death signalling, cytotoxicity or cellular apoptosis (Zhou et al., 2002). TNFR1 and TNFR2 compete for TNF-α (Bodmer et al., 2002). *TNFA* is instrumental in controlling and regulating viral infection, NF-κB signalling, neuropathic pain and cytokines (Lee et al., 2009). In the central nervous system (CNS), glial-derived *TNFA* modulates synaptic plasticity by increasing the expression of *AMPA* and also reducing long-term potentiation in the hippocampus (Leung and Cahill, 2010; Orlinick and Chao, 1998; Pickering et al., 2005). *TNFA* expression increases in the presence of stress and this has been observed in CFS patients although this increase was similar in healthy controls (Light et al., 2009). While mRNA levels in *TNFA* may be similar in CFS and healthy controls, polymorphism within *TNFA* may affect their ability to perform efficiently as shown in other diseases (Zhang et al., 2010).

IFNAR1 is required for IFNα/β antiviral responses and is therefore a key component in immunity against viral and bacterial infections (David, 2002). CFS patients are known to have significant increases in viral antigens and these may persist where the activities of IFNs are ineffective in inducing antiviral immune responses (Bansal et al., 2011). In CFS, *IFNAR1* is increased in expression (Kerr et al., 2008) and this may occur as a result of persistent viral antigens or viral infected cells. It has been observed that *IFNAR1* tends to increase in the presence of infections such as Human papillomavirus (HPV) and influenza (Gius et al., 2007; Jia et al., 2010). *IL10-RA* is both down- and up-regulated in CFS patients (Kaushik et al., 2005; Kerr et al., 2008). The protein, IL10-Rα is expressed on T cells, B cells, monocytes, macrophages, dendritic cells, NK cells, mast cells and microglia with no intrinsic kinase activity. Interactions between IL10-Rα and IL-10 stimulate the phosphorylation and activation of JAK1 and TYK2 kinases (Hebenstreit et al., 2005; O'Shea et al., 2002). This sequentially phosphorylates tyrosine residues in the cytoplasmic regions of IL-10Rα chains and forms docking sites for STAT3 (Moore et al., 2001). Janus Kinases and signal transducers and activators of transcription (JAK/STAT) pathways are essential for regulating cytokine mediated responses and *vice versa* (Schindler, 1999; Schindler et al., 2007). Genes such as *STAT5A* are induced by cytokines IL-2, IL-4 and IL-7. *STAT5A* is a critical element in the proliferation and survival of Th2 cells (Hebenstreit et al., 2005; Lin and Leonard, 2000). Differential expression in *STAT5A* in CFS likely affects the Th1-Th2 cytokine balance, possibly favouring an anti-inflammatory/Th1 like immune response, while suppressing pro-inflammatory immune reactions (Ihle, 2001; Kagami et al., 2001; Saiki et al., 2008; Skowera et al., 2004).

JAK1 contains cytoplasmic tyrosine kinases that react in a non-covalent manner to a varying number of cytokine receptors and is therefore implicated in lymphocyte development in particular, lymphocyte proliferation and differentiation (Flex et al., 2008). *STAT5A* and *JAK1* are requisite for IL-2, IL-10, IL-7, IL-9, IL-13, IL-22 and IFN-α signalling (Schindler et al.,

2007). Hence, over expression of both *STAT5A* and *JAK1* (Kerr et al., 2008; Saiki et al., 2008) may substantially alter the normal function of these cytokines and their receptors. These may include IFN-α, IL-7 and IL-10 (Kerr, 2008). Such adverse effects may cause shifts in the inflammatory profile causing either an increase or decrease in pro- and anti-inflammatory cytokines (Gupta et al., 1997; Vojdani et al., 1997). The exact profile of cytokines in CFS remains to be determined, although, a number of studies suggest that CFS is characterised by a predominant anti-inflammatory immune state (Skowera et al., 2004) others advocate a pro-inflammatory immune profile (Swanik et al.). This mixed picture suggests dysregulation of the balance in pro- and anti-inflammatory mechanisms.

Bidirectional communication between JAK/STAT signalling and cytokines is important for maintaining immune homeostasis. For example, IL-6 binds to its receptor and positively stimulates a number of JAKs and STATs which initiates a sequence of downstream effects that prompt the development and maturation of progenitor cells (Kamimura et al., 2003; Kristiansen and Mandrup-Poulsen, 2005). However, the expression of *IL-6* can be dampened by suppressors of cytokine signalling (SOCS), this inevitably increases inflammation (Croker et al., 2003; Zhang et al., 2008). Hence, differential expression in *IL-6, IL6R* and *IL6ST* (Kerr, 2008; Light et al., 2009) may have adverse consequences on the activity of IL-6 in both the innate and adaptive immune response. This may also affect *JAK1* in CFS (Guschin et al., 1995). Therefore in CFS differential expression in cytokine, JAK and STAT genes may increase susceptibility to prolonged immune deterioration.

TNFRSF1A is the gene for pro-inflammatory tumour necrosis factor (TNF)-α receptor, which increases pro-inflammatory events and stimulates the generation of cytokines through the activation of NF-κB (Nowlan et al., 2006). *TNFRSF1A* is also involved in cell death pathways involving TNFR-associated factor (TRAF) domains (Baud and Karin, 2001). In some CFS patients, cell death is particularly increased in neutrophils in comparison to non-fatigued controls (Kennedy et al., 2004; See et al., 1998; Vojdani et al., 1997). NF-κB gene, *NFKB1,* is decreased in expression in some CFS patients. Decreases in both *NFKB1* and *TNFRSF1A* in CFS may potentially affect the proliferation of cytokines and chemokines such as IL-8 (Kerr, 2008). Additionally, NF-κB is inhibited by *NFKBIZ* which is also down regulated in CFS (Kerr, 2008). In the immune system, NF-κB is activated in response to toll-like receptors (TLR) (Kitamura et al., 2000; Yamazaki et al., 2001) by *TRAF3* (Hauer et al., 2005; He et al., 2007; He et al., 2006). *TRAF3* is instrumental in T cell related immune responses (Goldfeld et al., 1991). *TRAF3* and *NFKBIZ* are collectively involved in the downstream activities of TNFRSF1A and NF-κB. Modifications in these genes can affect other cytokine pathways.

Another important gene, *HIF1A,* which encodes for the hypoxia induced transcription factor HIF1α, is responsible for the induction of apoptosis and inhibition of cell proliferation (Akakura et al., 2001; Carmeliet and Tessier-Lavigne, 2005; Yu et al., 2004). *HIF1A* also regulates pathogen lysis or phagocytosis mediated by neutrophils and macrophage (Nizet and Johnson, 2009). Oxidative phosphorylation is an important component of the phagolytic mechanism. This is deficient in some CFS cases and may cause a decrease in the amount of reactive oxygen species released from neutrophils to effectively breakdown the phagocytosed pathogen (Brenu et al. 2010). Impairments in oxidative phosphorylation in CFS patients may ensue from a downregulation in *HIF1A*.

As previously mentioned, chemokines such as IL-8 are important soluble proteins that are necessary for immune cell trafficking during infection and other inflammatory insults. Chemokines such as CXCR4 are expressed by neutrophils, monocytes and T lymphocytes and their activities are regulated by cAMP, IL-6, IL-4, IL-10 and reactive oxygen species (Jazin et al., 1997). CXCR4 is necessary for hematopoietic cell trafficking, differentiation, endothelial migration and cell proliferation in the CNS and immune systems (Jazin et al., 1997; Moepps et al., 1997; Zou et al., 1998). *CXCR4* is another gene involved in the identification of microbial factors such as LPS. The CXCR4 protein is part of the seven trans-membrane G-protein super family of receptors (Pierce et al., 2002). *CXCR4* promotes the proliferation of tumour cells via the MAP/ERK pathway and can in some cases have anti-apoptotic properties (Darash-Yahana et al., 2004). Similar to the *TLR4* and *CD14* in response to LPS, *CXCR4* expression becomes upregulated (Moriuchi et al., 1998). As these genes were simultaneously measured in the same CFS population, it is possible to posit that in some cases of CFS there are high levels of LPS factors, in particular LPS factors that cause heightened persistent immune activation. In these individuals perhaps these immune activations are not cleared and therefore encourage the survival of these microbial pathogens in circulation for a longer duration. In some CFS patients, *CXCR4* is upregulated (Gow et al., 2009; Kerr, 2008) which may suggest an altered chemokine profile in CFS patients. Other genes such as *CD47* are present on cells in the CNS and immune system. CD47 is a necessary factor in the migration of neutrophils and other cells (Brown et al., 1990; Gao et al., 1996; Lindberg et al., 1993; Parkos et al., 1996). It is also important in T cell activation and neurological function such as memory (Ticchioni et al., 1997; Waclavicek et al., 1997). In CFS, lymphocyte numbers in circulation may vary from patient to patient, however, the available number of lymphocytes at sites of infection or engaged in eliminating infected cells is not known. Incidentally, an upregulation in chemokine genes *IL-8*, *CXCR4* and *CD47* may affect the efficiency of these cells to migrate to areas of infection (Gow et al., 2009; Kerr, 2008).

As previously discussed *TGF-β1* is an important pleiotropic cytokine as it regulates peripheral tolerance mechanisms in response to injury, cell growth and survival (Marie et al., 2005). *TGF-β1* is a critical component of the Treg differentiation pathway in particular Treg survival and FOXP3 expression (Marie et al., 2005). *TGF-β1* is also an important factor in cellular apoptosis involving Fas mediated apoptotic pathways and oxidative phosphorylation (Sanchez-Capelo, 2005). An upregulation in this gene may stimulate pathways that increase spontaneous apoptosis in neutrophils (Kennedy et al., 2004) and thereby prevent the induction of oxidative stress in CFS individuals (Brenu et al., 2010).

2.4.2 Genes involved in pathogen lysis

An important mechanism employed by both NK and $CD8^+$T cells to lyse viral pathogens is cytotoxic activity. The end result of cytotoxicity is cell death or apoptosis. Cytotoxic activity is achieved when the NK or $CD8^+$T cells release lytic granules containing granzymes and perforin into the target cell through exocytosis (Leong & Fehinger 2010). In the cell membrane of the infected cell perforin facilitates the binding of granzymes to different organelles of the cell and induce either caspase dependent or independent apoptosis (Pradelli et al., 2010). *GZMA* is the gene for granzyme A, it is essential for natural cytotoxic activity and antibody dependent cytotoxic activity of $CD8^+$T and NK cells via FCγRII (CD16) receptor (Lahmers et al., 2006; Madueno et al., 1993). GZMA induces slow apoptosis once released into the target cell. In some CFS patients mRNA levels for *GZMA* and *GZMB* are low while levels of perforin are increased (Brenu et al., 2010; Saiki et al., 008). Differential expression in these lytic molecules may explain the inefficiency of NK or $CD8^+T$ cells in CFS patients to effectively execute cytotoxicity in the presence of pathogenic cells (Kilmas et al., 1990; Maher et al., 2005; Brenu et al., 2011).

However, discrepancies in the cathepsin C (*CTSC*) gene, which has wide distribution throughout the human body particularly in myeloid cells, polymorphonuclear leukocytes, alveolar macrophages and osteoclasts, can potentially affect the effectiveness of lytic cells (Hakeda and Kumegawa, 1991; McGuire et al., 1997; Rao et al., 1997b). Deficiencies in *CTSC* are associated with impaired activation of GZMA and GZMB in NK and cytotoxic T lymphocytes (Pham and Ley, 1999). This implies that CFS patients presenting with atypical *CTSC* expression may also exhibit decreased GZMA and GZMB production (Maher et al., 2005; Saiki et al., 2008). Cytotoxic activity may be considerably low as a consequence of low expression of granzyme genes in CFS patients, thus an increase in viral load will be highly detrimental to the compromised immune system.

2.4.3 Transcription factors

The regulation of genes is dependent on molecules known as transcription factors (Farnham, 2009). In CFS, transcription factor genes are differentially expressed. Among them is *EGR3,* which regulates lymphocyte proliferation, apoptosis and inflammatory responses (Beinke and Ley, 2004; Inoue et al., 2004; Jiang et al., 2005). *EGR3* in T lymphocytes stimulates Fas-L formation and cytotoxic activity of $CD8^+T$ lymphocytes (Matsuoka and Jeang, 2005). Their dysregulation affects the production of IL-2 (Safford et al., 2005), an important factor in anti-inflammatory Treg and Th2 differentiation. In CFS patients this may be associated with the deficits in cytotoxic activity and the presence of anti-inflammatory immune responses (Kerr et al., 2008).

TRAIL is another gene expressed by both innate and adaptive immune cells. It is important in inducing cellular apoptosis in immune cells, monocytes, dendritic cells, NK and $CD8^+T$ lymphocytes (Schaefer et al., 2007). In cytotoxic cells such as NK and $CD8^+T$, TRAIL serves as an alternative pathway for effective cytotoxic activity against viral antigens (Janssen et al., 2005; Kayagaki et al., 1999). Th2 cells preferentially express TRAIL and therefore are able to kill other immune cells and infected cells (Zhang et al., 2003). Hence, CFS patients with deficiencies in this gene may experience decreases in NK and $CD8^+T$ cell cytotoxic activity and induction of apoptosis, making them more vulnerable to immune infection and hindering normal immune function in these individuals.

NFATC1 is the gene for the nuclear factor of activated T lymphocytes belonging to the NFAT family of transcription factors. This transcription factor regulates genes encoding cytokines and cytokine receptors in response to antigen activation (Crabtree and Clipstone, 1994; Rao et al., 1997a). Importantly, they are implicated in T cell abundance, Th2 differentiation and cytokine production (Yoshida et al., 1998; Ranger et al., 1998). Impaired Th2 cytokines in some cases of CFS may emanate from perturbed expression in *NFATC1.* Conversely, other genes such as human β-defensin 1 *(DEFB1)* may have unfavourable consequences on the Th1 cytokines causing an over abundance of these proteins in some cases of CFS (Wehkamp et al., 2005). *DEFB1* is involved in immunomodulation against microbial peptides in both the innate and adaptive immune response. Using the CCR6 receptor they are able attract dendritic cells and CD4+T lymphocytes (Yang et al., 1999) during infection and inflammation (Dommisch et al., 2005; Sun et al., 2005; Wehkamp et al., 2005). Animal models have confirmed that an increase in susceptibility to microbial infections infections ensues in the event where *DEFB1* is deficient or mutated (Morrison et al., 2002; Moser et al., 2002). CFS related serological and virological studies indicate significant increases in viral antigens in some CFS patients and this may also be linked to defects in *DEFB1*.

ETS1 encodes for a transcription factor that binds to DNA sequences with an invariant GGA (Gegonne et al., 1993). *ETS1* like many other transcription factors is upregulated in CFS patients (Kerr et al., 2008). *ETS1* is an early response transcription factor gene with binding sites for transcription factors AP1, AP2 and ETS at its promoter end (Dittmer, 2003; Thomas et al., 1997). It is found in the nucleus where phosphorylation of Ras strongly increases transcriptional activity of ETS1 and its interactions with other proteins through the ETS1 domain (Wasylyk et al., 1998). *ETS1* acts together with other genes to increase its function hence it is positively regulated by AML-1, Pit-1 and HIF-2α (Dittmer, 2003). *ETS1* sequentially excites the DNA binding process of these genes . ETS1 can be inhibited by CAMKII, Daxx/EAPI and ZEB (Dittmer, 2003). ETS1 synergises with TGF-β to activate other genes. Activated T cells usually have a decreased expression of *ETS1* compared with dormant T cells T cells (Bhat et al., 1990). *ETS1* is found in T, B, and NK cells. It is a proto-oncogenic transcription factor which is involved in naïve T cell development and differentiation (Di Santo, 2010). In T cells, deficiencies in *ETS1* can inhibit T cell responses to other stimulatory signals and increase susceptibility to cell death. Although, *ETS1* expression decreases in the activated T cells in the developing T cell it is essential in prompting the expression of *TCRa* and *TCRβ* (Giese et al., 1995). Additionally, *ETS1* interacts with other immune regulators such as STAT5 which is implicated in T cell responses (Rameil et al., 2000). *ETS1* is an essential gene necessary for the optimal optimal development of naïve T cells, an increase in this gene may suggest an increase in resting T cells over activated T cells in CFS patients. Although, increases in some subsets of T cells such as FOXP3 Tregs (Brenu et al., 2011b) have been suggested, it is possible that these cells are not adequately activated and a majority of these cells are in the resting phase it is most likely thus are not able to effectively clear infections or encourage most favourable immune profile in CFS patients. NK decrease in cytotoxic activity may also be related to *ETS1* over expression as *ETS1* is important in NK cell development (Yokoyama et al., 2003). Failure of NK cells to develop into efficient lytic cells can hinder their ability to recognise and eliminate pathogens. Loss of function in ETS1 impairs proper lymphocyte differentiation and permits autoimmune responses (Wang et al., 2005). However, FOXN1 is involved in the development and differentiation of thymic epithelial cells (TECs) (Su et al., 2003). The expression of *FOXN1* is controlled by Bone Morphogenetic proteins (BMPs) and WNT (Coffer and Burgering, 2004). Immune deficiencies arise when mutations occur in *FOXN1* (Coffer and Burgering, 2004). In CFS, *FOXN1* has been suggested as a potential candidate gene for the development of biomarkers for CFS and may be linked to the severity of CFS (Presson et al., 2008). Abnormal changes in *FOXN1* affects T cell development and function and may relate to the cytokine pattern in CFS.

The histone acetyltransferase and deacetylase (*HDAC7A*) gene modulates nuclear histone acetylation. It inhibits the activity of myocyte enhancer-binding factor (MEF) and is highly expressed in thymocytes (Kasler and Verdin, 2007). This gene is responsible for transcriptional repression and the maintenance of cellular integrity (de Ruijter et al., 2003). It is an efficient co-repressor of the androgen receptor (AR) (Karvonen et al., 2006). It regulates apoptosis in developing thymocytes and may be associated with the decrease cytotoxic activity noticed in some CFS patients. Given that transcription factors are important in most cellular processes, a decrease or increase in its expression can have crucial consequences on the normal functioning of many physiological processes.

2.4.4 Immune regulators

The current data on CFS strongly support an impaired immune function characterised by differential expression of cytokines and decreases in cytotoxic activity. These observed immune defects may ensue from changes in the expression of certain genes involved in the signalling pathways of these immune indices. *MAPK9* codes an important signalling molecule known as the JNK2 protein kinase and its disruption is associated with the pathogenesis of destructive insulitis (Jaeschke et al., 2005). Some microbes are able to downregulate MAPK9 which in turn inactivates JNK2 thereby decreasing transcriptional events in this pathway (Zhang et al., 2004).

The cytochrome P450 (*CYPIBI*) gene has a role in responding to environmental toxins and mutagenic products (Hayes et al., 1996; Shimada et al., 1996). Although it is expressed in higher concentrations in breast cancer (Huang et al., 1996), in CFS it most likely involved in increased susceptibility to toxic agents. As CFS is likely a multi-factorial disorder, prolonged exposure to toxic agents may predispose an individual to CFS. *CMRF35/CD300C* encodes the CD300c leukocyte surface protein present on macrophages (Turnbull and Colonna, 2007). Secretion of TNF-α and IFN-α is highly dependent on *CYPIBI* (Ju et al., 2008). Additionally, abnormalities in CFS cytokine profiles possibly occurs where *CMRF35* is differentially expressed, distorting anti-viral (IFN- α) and pro-inflammatory (TNF-α) activities required for maintaining immune homeostasis (Sen, 2001).

Adhesion molecules are important for interactions between T cells and other cellular surfaces. In T cells the adhesion molecule CD2 allows T cells to connect with other cells. CD2 is regulated by *CD2BP2* (the CD2 binding protein 2) which increases binding specificity of the cytoplasmic domain of the T cell adhesion molecule CD2 and localizes it to the cell membrane and nucleus. TLR4 is an anti-tumour repressor and which inhibits the destruction of tumour antigens in lysosomes of dendritic cells. This facilitates antigen presentation to T cells and enhances the binding of LPS to MD-2. TLR4 mediated signalling can either occur via MyD88 dependent or independent pathway. When the MyD88 dependent pathway is used, this leads to the production of pro-inflammatory cytokines while the MyD88-independent pathway induces Type I interferons and interferon inducible genes (Lu et al., 2008). Human macrophages express CD14, a glycosylphosphatidylinositol-linked plasma-membrane glycoprotein, on their cell surfaces that facilitate the induction of apoptosis of foreign cells (Vita et al., 1997). *CD14* in conjunction with *TLR4* and *MD2* initiates the formation of a lipopolysaccharide receptor complex that controls immune responses to pathogens in the respiratory system, recognition of LPS and the generation of systemic inflammation (Wright et al., 1990). An increased expression in both *TLR4* and *CD14* may suggest an increase in LPS, LPS increases the expression of these genes (Foster et al., 2007). The biphasic expression of these genes allows them to have either an activating or a limiting effect on other genes. Additionally, in most cellular responses to bacterial infection due to LPS release, the MyD88-independent signalling pathway is activated. TLR4 may bind to the cell membrane allowing efficient presentation of LPS to TLR4. It is evident that modulation of the expression of *CD14* and *TLR4* can have severe consequences on the ability of immune cells to recognise microbial particles. Nonetheless, these observations are indicative of a heightened immune activation as a possible contributory factor to the compromised immune function in CFS patients.

Other neutrophil related genes have also been suggested to be differentially expressed in CFS patients. Genes such as *SNAP23* (Synaptosomal-associated protein 23) and *CFACAM8* are upregulated in some cases of CFS (Gow et al., 2009; Kerr et al., 2008). *SNAP23* is present mostly in non-neuronal tissues and is part of the t-SNARE complex (Washbourne et al., 2002). *SNAP23* controls neutrophil exocytosis and also cell surface granule interactions and is thus essential for intracellular trafficking of vesicles/granules (Lacy, 2006; Zylbersztejn and Galli, 2011). *CFACAM8* on the other hand is important in cell adhesion, migration and signal transduction in neutrophils (Zhao et al., 2004). These genes are therefore essential for the movement of neutrophils to sites of inflammation and or infection.

2.4.5 Other cellular processes

Other genes examined in CFS are necessary for many cellular processes. These genes may be implicated in functional properties of cells in a number of physiological processes suggesting a heterogeneous clinical presentation. For example, *ARPC5* is the smallest subunit of the actin related protein complex 5, which controls the polymerization of actin (Pollard, 2007). This normally occurs in response to cellular motility during the polymerization of new actin filament. Dendritic cells have not being adequately investigated in CFS, however, their morphogenesis may be compromised as evident by the over expression of *ANAPC11* (Gumy et al., 2011). *ANAPC11*, anaphase promoting complex subunit 11, has a role in dendritic cell morphogenesis (Domingo-Gil et al., 2010). It is part of a complex that targets and degrades proteins during mitosis. The migration of cells from one point to another, in circulation, involves the interplay of a number of genes such as *ATP5J2*, an ATP synthase involved in cellular processes requiring ATP (Cheung and Spielman, 2009). *APP*, the amyloid precursor gene is a marker for Alzheimer's disease (Zetterberg et al., 2010). It regulates cell surface proteins (Hoe and Rebeck, 2008).*GSN* is an anti-apoptotic regulator, and an actin serving protein that modulates actin assembly, disassembly and regulates cell motility via the actin network (Hoe and Rebeck, 2008). *REPIN1* is highly expressed in the liver and adipose tissue. It is a replication initiator and is involved in a number of metabolic disorders (Bahr et al., 2011).

A number of genes identified in CFS patients are involved in metabolic pathways specifically the protein kinases, ATP and cAMP related genes. These genes interact to maintain normal metabolic activity. These include transmembrane protein 50A (*TMEM50A)* located in RH gene locus, *ATP6V1C1* which regulates extracellular acidification to facilitate bone resorption (Feng et al., 2009) and *PRKAR1A* inhibits protein phosphorylation and tumour development (Bossis and Stratakis, 2004; Groussin et al., 2002). Mutations in *PRKAR1A* have been associated with tumour development (Scott, 1991; Tasken et al., 1997).

AKAP10 is the kinase-anchoring gene 10 which is currently an identifier for determining the risk of developing colorectal cancer (Wang et al., 2009a; Wang et al., 2009b). It also requires cAMP to diffuse through the cytoplasm to propagate its signal. *AKAP10* modulates immune responses related to PGE2/EP2/cAMP/PKA pathway (Kim et al., 2011). It targets regulatory subunit of PKA to specific cell sites such as the mitochondria. The cAMP responsive element binding protein (*CITED2)* refers to (Xu et al., 2007). It modulates hypoxia inducible factor dependent expression of vascular endothelial growth factor and hematopoietic stem cells. In CFS, we have recently reported an increase in neuropeptide receptors, specifically in VPACR2 in a cohort of CFS patients (Brenu et al., 2011b). This increase in VPAC2R may translate into an increase in cAMP causing a potential increase in PKA activity in CFS. An increase in cAMP may increase the expression of *PKAR1A, AKAP10* and *CITED2* and hence making their regulatory effects redundant and altering the physiological homeostasis. Tyrosine kinase non-receptor 2 (*TNK2)* functions as a translational repressor during cell fate specification and is necessary for the expression of epidermal growth factor receptors (Howlin et al., 2008).

Mitochondria related genes are also differentially expressed in CFS these genes include *SUCLA2, MRRF, EIF4G1, MRPL23, GABPA, PRDX3* and *EIF3S8*. As cellular function is impaired in CFS it is likely that important organelles especially those related to metabolic processing may be functioning at suboptimal levels. *SUCLA2*is involved in mitochondria regulation (Miller et al., 2011), *EIF4G1* is an initiation factor implicated in mitochondrial induced apoptosis (Bushell et al., 2000), *MRRF* regulates cell survival (Rorbach et al., 2008) while *PRDX3* prevents oxidative damage to cells (Ejima et al., 2000). Additionally, *GABPA, EIF3S8* and *MRPL23* have broad functions in mitochondria (Wyrwicz et al., 2007; Zhang and Wong-Riley, 2000). Mitochondria in the muscles of patients with CFS produce relatively low energy when compared to non-fatigued controls (Plioplys and Plioplys, 1995). In some cases patients may present with structural deformities in the mitochondria, these include subsarcolemmal mitochondrial aggregates, compartmentalization of the internal mitochondrial membrane and polymorphism (Plioplys and Plioplys, 1995). Similarly defective mitochondrial metabolic activity may be characterised by the presence of neurotoxic phospholipids and phospholipids of mitochondria that appear after microbial infections (Hokama et al., 2008). Neutrophil in the innate immune system employ respiratory burst and oxidative phosphorylation as a means to effectively kill and clear pathogen invasion. This unique mechanism is advantageous and reduces the persistence of microbial infections. Respiratory burst in CFS is flawed. The authors have previously shown that in CFS neutrophils are able to recognise and engulf pathogens however, the ability to induce and activate reactive oxygen species to induce respiratory burst is significantly compromised when compared to non-fatigued controls (Brenu et al., 2010). Incidentally, abnormal mitochondrial function exists in CFS where ATP and oxidative phosphorylation is substantially lower in the CFS patients (Myhill et al., 2009).

2.4.6 Neurology and endocrine function

Neurological dysfunction in CFS may present in many formats, the most obvious documented symptoms are loss in memory and concentration, sleep disorder and severe headaches. While the exact cause of CFS remains to be determined it has been postulated that neuroimmune abnormalities in form of dysregulation in cytokines due to a prevalent viral antigens in the brain may enhance CFS related neurological deficits (Kuratsune et al., 2001). In CFS a number of genes that regulate neurological and endocrine function have also being detected to be equivocally expressed when compared to non-fatigued controls. These observations may relate to the impairment in cognition and other neurological functions associated with this disease. The HPA axis is distorted in CFS and this may have a bearing on the changes in other genes (Ursini et al., 2010). EIF2B4 affects neurological function and has been shown to be related to mitochondrial function. It refers to the eukaryotic translation factor 2B subunit 4. It has been implicated in Vanishing White Matter disease (VWM). Although CFS is not an inherited disorder it may share similar symptoms with VWM. Both CFS and VWM are associated with infections (Bansal et al., 2011). CFS patients and patients with VWM may demonstrate abnormalities in cerebrospinal fluid (Schutzer et al., 2011a; Schutzer et al., 2011b). White matter studies in CFS are inconsistent, in some instances, abnormal white matter has been observed (Lange et al., 1999; Schwartz et al., 1994). Also, grey matter in some CFS patients may be reduced (de Lange et al., 2005). These confounding factors may to some extent relate to the severity of neurological impairments in patients with CFS.

NHLH1 is the helix-loop-helix transcription factor whose expression is restricted to the nervous system. It is important during development and neuronal differentiation (De Smaele et al., 2008). In mice loss of *NHLH1* generates irregular autonomic function characterised by arrhythmia, dampening of parasympathetic and in increase in death (Cogliati et al., 2002). A number of CFS patients may present with a dysfunctional autonomic system which may be related to an increase in heart rate and a decrease in systolic blood pressure. Additionally, irregularities in pH and heart rate variability occur in CFS patients following exercise (Jones et al., 2009; Newton et al., 2007). SORL1 refers to the sortilin-related receptor. It is a neuronal sorting protein-related receptor that is involved in intracellular trafficking. It directs trafficking of amyloid precursor protein and is decreased in the brains of humans suffering with Alzheimer's disease (Shibata et al., 2008). It is associated with risk of late onset of AD. This gene may be partially responsible for the memory loss experience by some CFS patients although this needs further clarification (Reynolds et al., 2010). *PKN1* is part of the neurofilament head rod domain kinase. It is a serine/threonine protein kinase that mediates cellular response to stress (Kato et al., 2008). *PKN1* regulates gene expression in response to extra cellular stimuli. Overexpression of *PKN1* causes a substantial elevation in the phosphorylation of ERK (Kajimoto et al., 2011). A number of CFS patients show an upregulation in genes in the ERK signalling pathway when compared to non-fatigue controls (Kerr et al., 2008). Phosphorylation of TRAF1 is dependent on *PNK1* and this also regulates the ratio of TRAF1 and TRAF2 and determines the NF-κβ and JNK signalling (Kat et al., 2008). TRAF1 and TRAF2 in turn modulate the signalling activity of IKK and JNK (Gotoh et al., 2004). An upregulation in *PKN1* may severely alter the downstream signalling pathways associated with PKN1. Importantly NF-κβ immune related activities maybe distorted where PKN1 is upregulated. NF- κβ regulates inflammatory cytokines (Park and Levitt, 1993). In CFS alterations in cytokine distribution has been observed. This may be either towards a pro- or anti-inflammatory cytokine profile. In the CNS system shifts in cytokine profiles have been reported for many autoimmune disorders and a similar mechanism may occur in CFS patients as a consequence of prevailing viral and microbial antigens that are not effectively cleared following infection. Perhaps these antigens remain and therefore modulate the cytokine milieu in the CNS.

Additionally heightened pro-inflammatory mechanisms followed by an increase in suppression may exist in the CNS neuroimmune system in an attempt to dampen viral and microbial survival in the CNS.

During development, *HOXA1* is expressed in the hindbrain (Studer et al., 1998). It is an essential developmental gene belonging to the homeobox genes. It is associated with autism. The product generated from translation of this gene is a transcription factor which is important in cell differentiation, embryogenesis, defining body plan during development and oncogenic transformation. Recently *HOXA1* has been observed to be a target of miR-10a (Shen et al., 2009). *COMT* is the catechol-O-methyltransferase, it is critical for the metabolic degradation of dopamine (Blanchard et al., 2011). It is involved in the function of dopamine in the prefrontal cortex of the human brain thus it is involved in frontal lobe functioning (Meyer-Lindenberg et al., 2005). The inability of most CFS patients to concentrate for long periods on activities requiring higher order cognitive function may be explained by dysregulation in *COMT*.

2.5 MicroRNA

MicroRNAs (miRNA) are recently described, highly conserved molecules with regulatory activities in multi-cellular organisms such as mammals. They are small components of ribonucleoprotein particles belonging to a family of RNA which have diverse effects on physiological function. MicroRNAs are suppressors of gene expression and affect either translational processes or the stability of mRNAs through the encouragement of decay processes, deadenylation and decapping processes termed RNA interference (Mishima et al., 2006; Wu et al., 2006). The expression of the miRNA gene results in the creation of the primary transcript (pri-miRNA) that is 60-80 nucleotides in length. This pri-miRNA contains a hairpin stem-loop structure which is cleaved by the enzyme Drosha (RNA III enzyme) and DGCR8 (DiGeorge critical region 8), resulting in the creation of a structure comprised of a ~22 base pair stem, 2-nucleotide 3′ overhang and a loop, collectively known as the precursor-miRNA (pre-miRNA) transcript (Lee et al., 2003). The pre-miRNA transcript is transported into the cytoplasm where RNase III enzyme, Dicer, cleaves the terminal loop of the pre-miRNA transcript to form a 18-24 base pair product (Lee et al., 2002). A currently unidentified helicase then produces individual miRNA strands - a mature miRNA, which is the mediator of mRNA repression, and the passenger strand, which is rapidly degraded. The mature miRNA is integrated into an RNA induced silencing complex (RISC) with Argonaute (Ago) proteins where it is further processed (Khvorova et al., 2003; Lee et al., 2003; Lingel et al., 2003; Mourelatos et al., 2002). The final product formed from this sequence of events is a miRNA-RISC complex. Suppressive effects of miRNA on mRNA molecules occur via the RISC complex in which Ago is able to exercise endonuclease activity on the double stranded miRNA-mRNA structure (Hutvagner and Zamore, 2002). The mature miRNA can bind to complete and incomplete complementary strands of mRNA molecules and degrade the mRNA or inhibit translation respectively (Behm-Ansmant et al., 2006; Hutvagner and Zamore, 2002; Lim et al., 2005). Through these mechanisms it has been extensively documented that miRNA regulates a diverse range of physiological activity and also contributes to disease states such as cancer (Lu et al., 2005) and cardiomyopathy (Chen et al., 2006). Interactions between the miRNA and mRNA molecules are important for maintaining physiological processes in development and homeostasis and have already been associated with numerous disease states. However, the role of miRNA in CFS is largely unknown. For further reading on the cellular and physiological processes of miRNA, the reader is directed to Sun et al. (2010).

With consistent trends between immunological dysfunction and CFS becoming more apparent, miRNAs related to immune function are relevant to this understudied area and may hold potential for treatment. The first study of its kind to assess miRNA expression in CFS investigated the expression of miRNAs relating to immune function, apoptosis and cell cycle regulation (Brenu et al., 2011a). This study identified a general down regulation in most of the miRNA transcripts in NK cells of CFS patients. This supports the observation of immune dysregulation in CFS patients (Brenu et al., 2010; Maher et al., 2005), however, whether this is linked to a decrease in miRNA processing activity or is specific to miRNA function is yet to be determined. More specifically, this study found decreases in miRNA transcripts that are involved in apoptosis. CFS patients have been shown to demonstrate significant decrease in cytotoxic activity of NK cells hence decreases in miRNAs may contribute to the pattern of NK cytotoxicity noticed in CFS patients. For example, miR-146, which mediates the expression of NFκ-β and thus the transcription of numerous inflammatory mediators, was significantly decreased in CFS (Brenu et al., 2011b). The consequence of this may be a decrease in the cytokine secretion by NK cells as NFκ-β is an important regulator of cytokine production in these cells (Gerondakis & Siebenlist 2010). Incidentally *IFN-γ* was noticed to be significantly decreased in expression in the same cohort of CFS patients with a decrease in miR-146 (Brenu et al., 2011b). Similarly, in the presence of an altered NFκB expression, NK responsiveness to IL-12 in CFS patients may be dampened compromising immune response to both infection and homeostasis (Broderick et al., 2010). Further studies are needed to verify whether miRNAs contribute or are linked to depressions in IL-8, IL-13 and IL-5 and increased activity of IL-1α, IL-1β, IL-4, IL-5, IL-6 and IL-12 in CFS patients (Fletcher et al., 2009). Substantial decreases in the expression miR-21 were observed in the CFS patient group. These results suggest the presence of a possible compromise in the maturation and function of lymphocyte translating into decreases in cytotoxic activity (Salaun et al., 2011). Direct evidence of this however, remains to be established.

At the present miRNA research is at its infancy hence the exact role of miRNAs in NK cells is subject to speculation. Similarly the gene expression miRNA studies in CFS is severely lacking therefore only postulations can be made about the link between the miRNAs and the disease. However, the promising data shown in the aforementioned studies likely suggest that miRNAs may indeed play greater roles in the dysregulation of immune function in CFS.

MicroRNAs may regulate other aspects of immune function in CFS, the above mentioned study is limited as it only examines NK and $CD8^{+}$T cells. However miRNAs are known to regulate most if not all immune cells. In the innate immune system, miRNAs such as miR-155 enhance the maturation of macrophages and dendritic cells via the TLR receptor pathway, causing heightened sensitivity in these cells to antigens in circulation (O'Connell et al., 2007; Tili et al., 2007). $CD4^{+}$ T cell matuation into various subsets in the periphery is regulated by miRNAs (Wu et al., 2007). The generation of Tregs that express FOXP3 is to some extent dependent on miRNAs (Kohlhaas et al., 2009). Any perturbed effects in miRNAs can influence thymic and peripheral derived Tregs especially in response to TGF-β stimulation on naive

$CD4^+$ T lymphocytes (Ha, 2011). Modulation of the effects of these molecules is essential for appropriate immune response to bacterial and viral invasion and current studies show these areas may be impaired in CFS sufferers. Importantly, deficiencies in components of the miRNA such as Dicer promotes a predominant Th1 response governed by IFN-γ with a reduction in the effects of Th2 cells and Treg cells (Cobb et al., 2006). In contrast a predominant Th2 $CD4^+$ T cell profile prompting systemic inflammation emanates from deficiencies in the miR-155 (Rodriguez et al., 2007; Thai et al., 2007) while in the absence of miR-101, autoreactive T cell mediated autoimmunity occurs (Yu et al., 2007). In CFS there are inconsistencies in the data on Th1/Th2 profiles. It is likely that in the event that immune related miRNAs are differentially expressed, shifts in Th1 and Th2 inflammatory response and defects in TLR signalling may occur, and this may be related to the pathophysiology of CFS. Whilst it is believed that many miRNAs are yet to be discovered, evidence is scarce to describe the multitude of various physiological roles of currently discovered miRNAs. Despite this, the current evidence that links miRNA dysregulation to the characteristics of CFS has shown that there is merit in the roles of miRNA in CFS. Further advancements are needed to characterise the role of miRNAs in CFS.

Our current investigative techniques for identifying transcriptional changes in known miRNAs are quickly advancing through microarray technology. This method uses the same principle as DNA microarray technology and allows for semi-quantitative expression changes of a large number of miRNAs in a single chip (Li and Ruan, 2009). The clear advantages of using microarray is the high throughput and vast number of transcripts analysed in a single chip as compared to low throughput and tedious methods of microRNA cloning, northern blotting and real time RT-qPCR. As mentioned in section 2.2, this gives investigators the power to identify expression differentials in gene categories, allowing the association of a particular state or disease to a molecular or physiological category. Numerous limitations are associated with microarray technology, most importantly is the ability to identify changes in already known miRNAs, as the targets require hybridisation with specifically designed probes attached to the chip. Moreover, these expression changes are only semi-quantitative due to the hybridisation techniques used, resulting in a lack of reproducibility. These pitfalls are similar to those in DNA microarray but are likely not as pronounced due to the various isoforms and large size of genes as compared with miRNAs (Fathallah-Shaykh, 2005). Finally, microarray technology has the disadvantage of only being able to detect known transcripts. With possibly many undiscovered transcripts this poses a problem for miRNA discovery in differential expression using this method and may also interfere with target specificity. However, more recent investigative techniques look promising for the discovery of new target miRNAs as well as addressing many of the pitfalls of the low-throughput and microarray based methods. One such example is sequence-by-synthesis technology, which has recently been used with investigative application and is likely to be used more widely in the near future (Morin et al., 2008).

2.6 MicroRNA-based gene therapy

The roles of microRNAs in diseases are likely to become targets for therapy. The current experimental practice is known as gene silencing and the specialised transcripts used in such instances are known as small interfering RNA (siRNA) (Wang et al., 2011). The cellular method of translation or transcription repression is the same as miRNAs – through the use of RISC, however in gene silencing the target-specific substrate, the siRNA, is exogenously introduced. There is currently little in the way of clinically translated practice of gene therapy using the siRNA method, as it is associated with a number of problems. The most notable of these is delivery and cell specific targeting. The current means of delivery in experimental models is via adeno- or adeno-associated virus constructs transcribing the specific siRNA or siRNAs of choice. To allow for cell specific targeting certain virus constructs are suited for various cell types however the lack of specificity and low percentage uptake makes this is an improbable method of therapy at present. There are however new experimental means of delivery currently being optimised (Yuan et al., 2011). Once such issues have been addressed the significance of gene silencing may be relevant in CFS. With increasing amounts of evidence indicating that CFS likely has a strong molecular basis, such methods hold merit once initial targets have been discovered. The current stance on miRNAs in CFS calls for further research in the area in both genome wide miRNA analysis in longitudinal studies, and also the search for new miRNAs possibly implicated in this disorder. With the current technology available, and promising experimental therapeutics such as gene silencing, miRNA is likely to play a large and significant role in possibly the development of biomarkers, mechanisms or treatment of CFS.

2.7 Future directions

The high variability in genomic anomalies within CFS patients may be an underlying cause of our current inability to effectively treat the disorder. No specific conditioning or dieting routine has proven beneficial for a wide majority of patients and even more elusive are effective pharmacological targets for this population. It is probable that various underlying mechanisms may give rise to the variable patient-described symptoms of CFS. This may explain the lack of efficient treatment options and opens questions in the area of pharmacogenomics. Pharmacological agents specific to genetic traits that are associated with CFS and possibly subsets of the disease may be useful in monitoring CFS. In the context of CFS, this pertains to our lack of understanding and inability to define areas of treatment, suggesting that a suitable treatment may call for the definition of subtypes of the disease or populations that are genetically predisposed to such symptoms.

However, at present the most important aim of research worldwide is to establish biomarkers for CFS. Currently the most stable and reliable marker is NK cytotoxic activity (Brenu et al., 2011b; Fletcher et al., 2009; Klimas et al., 1990; Maher et al., 2005). Consistent data worldwide suggest that a decrease in cytotoxic activity is a hallmark of CFS. In most cases this decrease has been associated with differential expression in cytotoxic molecules including *GZMA, GZMK, GZMB* and *PRF1* (Brenu et al., 2011b; Saiki et al., 2008). Developing pharmacological agents that specifically target these cytotoxic genes in order to increase or decrease their expression might be an alternative method of treating impaired cytotoxic activity in CFS patients. Subtypes of CFS patients may exist and this may be based on clusters of symptoms or severity of illness. Hence these may need to be considered when developing appropriate agents for modulating the disease.

3. Conclusion

In summary, the repercussions of these changes gene expresseion may contribute tremendously to the disease profile of CFS. The genes discussed above have vital roles in most immune related activities such as inflammatory modulation, lymphocyte and cytokine activation, lymphocyte differentiation and proliferation and are also implicated in the apoptosis signalling pathways. Hence, an up-regulation in chemokine genes may affect leukocyte response to infection and other immunological insults while down-regulation in pro-inflammatory cytokine genes may disrupt inflammatory reactions. Importantly, the consistent observation of impaired NK cytolysis in CFS is partly due to the reduced expression of perforin and granzymes genes. As previously discussed these granzymes induce apoptosis of antigens within the cell. Variation in cytokine release and production can be explained by the altered levels of pro- and anti-inflammatory cytokines. Most of these cytokines are engaged in other physiological processes. Hence, defects in their production can severely hinder physiological function and homeostasis. Other symptoms such as cognitive impairment and changes in the HPA axis in CFS patients may emanate from an increase *NHLH1* while changes in mitochondria genes contribute to fatigue and muscle weakness. Although, these studies have to some extent provided information on the genetics of CFS patients, it is not known whether CFS elicits these changes in gene expression patterns or *vice versa*. Similarly, most of the genes observed in these studies have not been replicated in other CFS patients. It is therefore very difficult to ascertain which specific cells are compromised among the CFS population. Further studies are now required to determine how changes in gene expression can be related to the mechanism of CFS and the specific cells or systems that may be severely compromised in this disorder.

4. References

Akakura, N., Kobayashi, M., Horiuchi, I., Suzuki, A., Wang, J., Chen, J., Niizeki, H., Kawamura, K., Hosokawa, M. and Asaka, M. (2001) Constitutive expression of hypoxia-inducible factor-1alpha renders pancreatic cancer cells resistant to apoptosis induced by hypoxia and nutrient deprivation. Cancer Res 61, 6548-54.

Albright, F., Light, K., Light, A., Bateman, L. and Cannon-Albright, L.A. (2011) Evidence for a heritable predisposition to Chronic Fatigue Syndrome. BMC Neurol 11, 62.

Arango, V., Huang, Y.Y., Underwood, M.D. and Mann, J.J. (2003) Genetics of the serotonergic system in suicidal behavior. Journal of psychiatric research 37, 375-86.

Artis, D., Speirs, K., Joyce, K., Goldschmidt, M., Caamano, J., Hunter, C.A. and Scott, P. (2003) NF-kappa B1 is required for optimal $CD4^+$ Th1 cell development and resistance to Leishmania major. J Immunol 170, 1995-2003.

Bahr, J., Kloting, N., Kloting, I. and Follak, N. (2011) Gene expression profiling supports the role of Repin1 in the pathophysiology of metabolic syndrome. Endocrine.

Bansal, A.S., Bradley, A.S., Bishop, K.N., Kiani-Alikhan, S. and Ford, B. (2011) Chronic fatigue syndrome, the immune system and viral infection. Brain Behav Immun.

Baud, V. and Karin, M. (2001) Signal transduction by tumor necrosis factor and its relatives. Trends Cell Biol 11, 372-7.

Behm-Ansmant, I., Rehwinkel, J. and Izaurralde, E. (2006) MicroRNAs silence gene expression by repressing protein expression and/or by promoting mRNA decay. Cold Spring Harb Symp Quant Biol 71, 523-30.

Beinke, S. and Ley, S.C. (2004) Functions of NF-kappaB1 and NF-kappaB2 in immune cell biology. The Biochemical journal 382, 393-409.

Bellone, G., Aste-Amezaga, M., Trinchieri, G. and Rodeck, U. (1995) Regulation of NK cell functions by TGF-beta 1. J Immunol 155, 1066-73.

Bhat, N.K., Thompson, C.B., Lindsten, T., June, C.H., Fujiwara, S., Koizumi, S., Fisher, R.J. and Papas, T.S. (1990) Reciprocal expression of human ETS1 and ETS2 genes during T-cell activation: regulatory role for the protooncogene ETS1. Proc Natl Acad Sci U S A 87, 3723-7.

Blanchard, M.M., Chamberlain, S.R., Roiser, J., Robbins, T.W. and Muller, U. (2011) Effects of two dopamine-modulating genes (DAT1 9/10 and COMT Val/Met) on n-back working memory performance in healthy volunteers. Psychol Med 41, 611-8.

Bodmer, J.L., Schneider, P. and Tschopp, J. (2002) The molecular architecture of the TNF superfamily. Trends Biochem Sci 27, 19-26.

Bohuslav, J., Kravchenko, V.V., Parry, G.C., Erlich, J.H., Gerondakis, S., Mackman, N. and Ulevitch, R.J. (1998) Regulation of an essential innate immune response by the p50 subunit of NF-kappaB. J Clin Invest 102, 1645-52.

Bossis, I. and Stratakis, C.A. (2004) Minireview: PRKAR1A: normal and abnormal functions. Endocrinology 145, 5452-8.

Brenu, E.W., Ashton, K.J., van Driel, M., Staines, D.R., Peterson, D., Atkinson, G.M. and Marshall-Gradisnik, S.M. (2011a) MicroRNAs Analysis in Cytotoxic Lymphocytes of Chronic Fatigue Syndrome/Myalgic Encephalomyelitis Patients. BMC Immunology.

Brenu, E.W., Staines, D.R., Baskurt, O.K., Ashton, K.J., Ramos, S.B., Christy, R.M. and Marshall-Gradisnik, S.M. (2010) Immune and hemorheological changes in chronic fatigue syndrome. Journal of translational medicine 8, 1.

Brenu, E.W., van Driel, M.L., Staines, D.R., Ashton, K.J., Ramos, S.B., Keane, J., Klimas, N.G. and Marshall-Gradisnik, S.M. (2011b) Immunological abnormalities as potential biomarkers in Chronic Fatigue Syndrome/Myalgic Encephalomyelitis. Journal of translational medicine 9, 81.

Bright, J.J., Kerr, L.D. and Sriram, S. (1997) TGF-beta inhibits IL-2-induced tyrosine phosphorylation and activation of Jak-1 and Stat 5 in T lymphocytes. J Immunol 159, 175-83.

Brkic, S., Tomic, S., Ruzic, M. and Maric, D. (2011) Chronic fatigue syndrome. Srpski arhiv za celokupno lekarstvo 139, 256-61.

Broderick, G., Fuite, J., Kreitz, A., Vernon, S.D., Klimas, N. and Fletcher, M.A. (2010) A formal analysis of cytokine networks in chronic fatigue syndrome. Brain, behavior, and immunity 24, 1209-17.

Brown, E., Hooper, L., Ho, T. and Gresham, H. (1990) Integrin-associated protein: a 50-kD plasma membrane antigen physically and functionally associated with integrins. J Cell Biol 111, 2785-94.

Buchwald, D., Herrell, R., Ashton, S., Belcourt, M., Schmaling, K., Sullivan, P., Neale, M. and Goldberg, J. (2001) A twin study of chronic fatigue. Psychosom Med 63, 936-43.

Bushell, M., Wood, W., Clemens, M.J. and Morley, S.J. (2000) Changes in integrity and association of eukaryotic protein synthesis initiation factors during apoptosis. Eur J Biochem 267, 1083-91.

Cameron, B., Galbraith, S., Zhang, Y., Davenport, T., Vollmer-Conna, U., Wakefield, D., Hickie, I., Dunsmuir, W., Whistler, T., Vernon, S., Reeves, W.C. and Lloyd, A.R. (2007) Gene expression correlates of postinfective fatigue syndrome after infectious mononucleosis. J Infect Dis 196, 56-66.

Campbell, I.K., Gerondakis, S., O'Donnell, K. and Wicks, I.P. (2000) Distinct roles for the NF-kappaB1 (p50) and c-Rel transcription factors in inflammatory arthritis. J Clin Invest 105, 1799-806.

Carlo-Stella, N., Bozzini, S., De Silvestri, A., Sbarsi, I., Pizzochero, C., Lorusso, L., Martinetti, M. and Cuccia, M. (2009) Molecular study of receptor for advanced glycation endproduct gene promoter and identification of specific HLA haplotypes possibly involved in chronic fatigue syndrome. Int J Immunopathol Pharmacol 22, 745-54.

Carlson, M.E., Hsu, M. and Conboy, I.M. (2008) Imbalance between pSmad3 and Notch induces CDK inhibitors in old muscle stem cells. Nature 454, 528-32.

Carmel, L., Efroni, S., White, P.D., Aslakson, E., Vollmer-Conna, U. and Rajeevan, M.S. (2006) Gene expression profile of empirically delineated classes of unexplained chronic fatigue. Pharmacogenomics 7, 375-86.

Carmeliet, P. and Tessier-Lavigne, M. (2005) Common mechanisms of nerve and blood vessel wiring. Nature 436, 193-200.

Carruthers, B.M., van de Sande, M.I., De Meirleir, K.L., Klimas, N.G., Broderick, G., Mitchell, T., Staines, D., Powles, A.P., Speight, N., Vallings, R., Bateman, L., Baumgarten-Austrheim, B., Bell, D.S., Carlo-Stella, N., Chia, J., Darragh, A., Jo, D., Lewis, D., Light, A.R., Marshall-Gradisbik, S., Mena, I., Mikovits, J.A., Miwa, K., Murovska, M., Pall, M.L. and Stevens, S. (2011) Myalgic Encephalomyelitis: International Consensus Criteria. Journal of internal medicine.

Carruthers, B.M., Jain, A.K., de Meirleir, K.L., Peterson, D.L., Klimas, N.G., Lerner, M., Bested, A.C., Flor-Henry, P., Joshi, P., Powles, A.C.P., Sherkey, J.A. & van de Sande, M.I. (2003) Myalgic Encephalomyelitis/Chronic Fatigue Syndrome:Clinical Working Case Definition, Diagnostic and Treatment Protocols. Journal of Chronic Fatigue, 11, 7-154.

Chen, J.F., Mandel, E.M., Thomson, J.M., Wu, Q., Callis, T.E., Hammond, S.M., Conlon, F.L. and Wang, D.Z. (2006) The role of microRNA-1 and microRNA-133 in skeletal muscle proliferation and differentiation. Nature genetics 38, 228-33.

Cheung, V.G. and Spielman, R.S. (2009) Genetics of human gene expression: mapping DNA variants that influence gene expression. Nat Rev Genet 10, 595-604.

Choy, L., Skillington, J. and Derynck, R. (2000) Roles of autocrine TGF-beta receptor and Smad signaling in adipocyte differentiation. J Cell Biol 149, 667-82.

Claypoole, K.H., Noonan, C., Mahurin, R.K., Goldberg, J., Erickson, T. and Buchwald, D. (2007) A twin study of cognitive function in chronic fatigue syndrome: the effects of sudden illness onset. Neuropsychology 21, 507-13.

Cobb, B.S., Hertweck, A., Smith, J., O'Connor, E., Graf, D., Cook, T., Smale, S.T., Sakaguchi, S., Livesey, F.J., Fisher, A.G. and Merkenschlager, M. (2006) A role for Dicer in immune regulation. J Exp Med 203, 2519-27.

Coffer, P.J. and Burgering, B.M. (2004) Forkhead-box transcription factors and their role in the immune system. Nat Rev Immunol 4, 889-99.

Cogliati, T., Good, D.J., Haigney, M., Delgado-Romero, P., Eckhaus, M.A., Koch, W.J. and Kirsch, I.R. (2002) Predisposition to arrhythmia and autonomic dysfunction in Nhlh1-deficient mice. Mol Cell Biol 22, 4977-83.

Crabtree, G.R. and Clipstone, N.A. (1994) Signal transmission between the plasma membrane and nucleus of T lymphocytes. Annu Rev Biochem 63, 1045-83.

Crawley, E. and Smith, G.D. (2207) Is Chronic Fatigue Syndrome (CFS/ME) heritable in children, and if so, why does it matter? Arch Dis Child 92, 1058-1061.

Croker, B.A., Krebs, D.L., Zhang, J.G., Wormald, S., Willson, T.A., Stanley, E.G., Robb, L., Greenhalgh, C.J., Forster, I., Clausen, B.E., Nicola, N.A., Metcalf, D., Hilton, D.J., Roberts, A.W. and Alexander, W.S. (2003) SOCS3 negatively regulates IL-6 signaling in vivo. Nat Immunol 4, 540-5.

Darash-Yahana, M., Pikarsky, E., Abramovitch, R., Zeira, E., Pal, B., Karplus, R., Beider, K., Avniel, S., Kasem, S., Galun, E. and Peled, A. (2004) Role of high expression levels of CXCR4 in tumor growth, vascularization, and metastasis. FASEB J 18, 1240-2.

David, M. (2002) Signal transduction by type I interferons. Biotechniques Suppl, 58-65.

de Lange, F.P., Kalkman, J.S., Bleijenberg, G., Hagoort, P., van der Meer, J.W. and Toni, I. (2005) Gray matter volume reduction in the chronic fatigue syndrome. Neuroimage 26, 777-81.

de Ruijter, A.J., van Gennip, A.H., Caron, H.N., Kemp, S. and van Kuilenburg, A.B. (2003) Histone deacetylases (HDACs): characterization of the classical HDAC family. Biochem J 370, 737-49.

De Smaele, E., Fragomeli, C., Ferretti, E., Pelloni, M., Po, A., Canettieri, G., Coni, S., Di Marcotullio, L., Greco, A., Moretti, M., Di Rocco, C., Pazzaglia, S., Maroder, M., Screpanti, I., Giannini, G. and Gulino, A. (2008) An integrated approach identifies Nhlh1 and Insm1 as Sonic Hedgehog-regulated genes in developing cerebellum and medulloblastoma. Neoplasia 10, 89-98.

Delvig, A.A., Lee, J.J., Chrzanowska-Lightowlers, Z.M. and Robinson, J.H. (2002) TGF-beta1 and IFN-gamma cross-regulate antigen presentation to CD4 T cells by macrophages. J Leukoc Biol 72, 163-6.

Demitrack, M.A. (1997) Neuroendocrine correlates of chronic fatigue syndrome: a brief review. J Psychiatr Res 31, 69-82.

Derynck, R. and Zhang, Y.E. (2003) Smad-dependent and Smad-independent pathways in TGF-beta family signalling. Nature 425, 577-84.

Dittmer, J. (2003) The biology of the Ets1 proto-oncogene. Mol Cancer 2, 29.

Domingo-Gil, E., Gonzalez, J.M. and Esteban, M. (2010) Identification of cellular genes induced in human cells after activation of the OAS/RNaseL pathway by vaccinia virus recombinants expressing these antiviral enzymes. J Interferon Cytokine Res 30, 171-88.

Dommisch, H., Acil, Y., Dunsche, A., Winter, J. and Jepsen, S. (2005) Differential gene expression of human beta-defensins (hBD-1, -2, -3) in inflammatory gingival diseases. Oral Microbiol Immunol 20, 186-90.

Ejima, K., Nanri, H., Araki, M., Koji, T., Shibata, E., Kashimura, M. and Ikeda, M. (2000) Expression of mitochondrial thioredoxin-dependent antioxidant protein, SP-22, in normal human and inflammatory mouse placentae. Placenta 21, 847-52.

Evengard, B., Jacks, A., Pedersen, N.L. and Sullivan, P.F. (2005) The epidemiology of chronic fatigue in the Swedish Twin Registry. Psychol Med 35, 1317-26.

Fang, H., Xie, Q., Boneva, R., Fostel, J., Perkins, R. and Tong, W. (2006) Gene expression profile exploration of a large dataset on chronic fatigue syndrome. Pharmacogenomics 7, 429-40.

Farnham, P.J. (2009) Insights from genomic profiling of transcription factors. Nat Rev Genet 10, 605-16.

Fathallah-Shaykh, H.M. (2005) Microarrays: applications and pitfalls. Archives of neurology 62, 1669-72.

Feng, S., Deng, L., Chen, W., Shao, J., Xu, G. and Li, Y.P. (2009) Atp6v1c1 is an essential component of the osteoclast proton pump and in F-actin ring formation in osteoclasts. Biochem J 417, 195-203.

Fletcher, M.A., Zeng, X.R., Barnes, Z., Levis, S. and Klimas, N.G. (2009) Plasma cytokines in women with chronic fatigue syndrome. Journal of translational medicine 7, 96.

Flex, E., Petrangeli, V., Stella, L., Chiaretti, S., Hornakova, T., Knoops, L., Ariola, C., Fodale, V., Clappier, E., Paoloni, F., Martinelli, S., Fragale, A., Sanchez, M., Tavolaro, S., Messina, M., Cazzaniga, G., Camera, A., Pizzolo, G., Tornesello, A., Vignetti, M., Battistini, A., Cave, H., Gelb, B.D., Renauld, J.C., Biondi, A., Constantinescu, S.N., Foa, R. and Tartaglia, M. (2008) Somatically acquired JAK1 mutations in adult acute lymphoblastic leukemia. J Exp Med 205, 751-8.

Foster, N., Lea, S.R., Preshaw, P.M. and Taylor, J.J. (2007) Pivotal advance: vasoactive intestinal peptide inhibits up-regulation of human monocyte TLR2 and TLR4 by LPS and differentiation of monocytes to macrophages. J Leukoc Biol 81, 893-903.

Fukuda, K., Straus, S.E., Hickie, I., Sharpe, M.C., Dobbins, J.G. and Komaroff, A. (1994) The chronic fatigue syndrome: a comprehensive approach to its definition and study. International Chronic Fatigue Syndrome Study Group. Ann Intern Med, 121, 953-9.

Gao, A.G., Lindberg, F.P., Finn, M.B., Blystone, S.D., Brown, E.J. and Frazier, W.A. (1996) Integrin-associated protein is a receptor for the C-terminal domain of thrombospondin. J Biol Chem 271, 21-4.

Gegonne, A., Bosselut, R., Bailly, R.A. and Ghysdael, J. (1993) Synergistic activation of the HTLV1 LTR Ets-responsive region by transcription factors Ets1 and Sp1. EMBO J 12, 1169-78.

Gerondakis, S. and Siebenlist, U. (2010) Roles of the NF-kappaB pathway in lymphocyte development and function. Cold Springs Harb Perspect Biol 2, a000182.

Giese, K., Kingsley, C., Kirshner, J.R. and Grosschedl, R. (1995) Assembly and function of a TCR alpha enhancer complex is dependent on LEF-1-induced DNA bending and multiple protein-protein interactions. Genes Dev 9, 995-1008.

Goldfeld, A.E., Strominger, J.L. and Doyle, C. (1991) Human tumor necrosis factor alpha gene regulation in phorbol ester stimulated T and B cell lines. J Exp Med 174, 73-81.

Gotoh, Y., Oishi, K., Shibata, H., Yamagiwa, A., Isagawa, T., Nishimura, T., Goyama, E., Takahashi, M., Mukai, H. and Ono, Y. (2004) Protein kinase PKN1 associates with TRAF2 and is involved in TRAF2-NF-kappaB signaling pathway. Biochem Biophys Res Commun 314, 688-94.

Gow, J.W., Hagan, S., Herzyk, P., Cannon, C., Behan, P.O. and Chaudhuri, A. (2009) A gene signature for post-infectious chronic fatigue syndrome. BMC medical genomics 2, 38.

Gros, M.J., Naquet, P. and Guinamard, R.R. (2008) Cell intrinsic TGF-beta 1 regulation of B cells. J Immunol 180, 8153-8.

Groussin, L., Kirschner, L.S., Vincent-Dejean, C., Perlemoine, K., Jullian, E., Delemer, B., Zacharieva, S., Pignatelli, D., Carney, J.A., Luton, J.P., Bertagna, X., Stratakis, C.A. and Bertherat, J. (2002) Molecular analysis of the cyclic AMP-dependent protein kinase A (PKA) regulatory subunit 1A (PRKAR1A) gene in patients with Carney complex and primary pigmented nodular adrenocortical disease (PPNAD) reveals novel mutations and clues for pathophysiology: augmented PKA signaling is associated with adrenal tumorigenesis in PPNAD. Am J Hum Genet 71, 1433-42.

Gu, T.L., Goetz, T.L., Graves, B.J. and Speck, N.A. (2000) Auto-inhibition and partner proteins, core-binding factor beta (CBFbeta) and Ets-1, modulate DNA binding by CBFalpha2 (AML1). Mol Cell Biol 20, 91-103.

Guis, D., Funk M.C., Chuang, E.Y., Feng, S., Huettner, P.C., Nguyen, L., Bradbury, C.M., Mishra, M., Gao, S., Buttin, B.M., Cohn, D.E., Powell, M.A., Horowitz, N.S., Whitcomb, B.P., Rader, J.S. (2007) Profiling microdissected epithelium and stroma to model genomic signatures for cervical carcinogenesis accommodating for covariates. Cancer Res 67, 7113-7123.

Gumy, L.F., Yeo, G.S., Tung, Y.C., Zivraj, K.H., Willis, D., Coppola, G., Lam, B.Y., Twiss, J.L., Holt, C.E. and Fawcett, J.W. (2011) Transcriptome analysis of embryonic and adult sensory axons reveals changes in mRNA repertoire localization. RNA 17, 85-98.

Gupta, S., Aggarwal, S., See, D. and Starr, A. (1997) Cytokine production by adherent and non-adherent mononuclear cells in chronic fatigue syndrome. J Psychiatr Res 31, 149-56.

Guschin, D., Rogers, N., Briscoe, J., Witthuhn, B., Watling, D., Horn, F., Pellegrini, S., Yasukawa, K., Heinrich, P., Stark, G.R. and et al. (1995) A major role for the protein tyrosine kinase JAK1 in the JAK/STAT signal transduction pathway in response to interleukin-6. EMBO J 14, 1421-9.

Ha, T.Y. (2011) The Role of MicroRNAs in Regulatory T Cells and in the Immune Response. Immune Netw 11, 11-41.

Hakeda, Y. and Kumegawa, M. (1991) [Osteoclasts in bone metabolism]. Kaibogaku Zasshi 66, 215-25.

Hauer, J., Puschner, S., Ramakrishnan, P., Simon, U., Bongers, M., Federle, C. and Engelmann, H. (2005) TNF receptor (TNFR)-associated factor (TRAF) 3 serves as an inhibitor of TRAF2/5-mediated activation of the noncanonical NF-kappaB pathway by TRAF-binding TNFRs. Proc Natl Acad Sci U S A 102, 2874-9.

Hayes, C.L., Spink, D.C., Spink, B.C., Cao, J.Q., Walker, N.J. and Sutter, T.R. (1996) 17 beta-estradiol hydroxylation catalyzed by human cytochrome P450 1B1. Proc Natl Acad Sci U S A 93, 9776-81.

He, J.Q., Saha, S.K., Kang, J.R., Zarnegar, B. and Cheng, G. (2007) Specificity of TRAF3 in its negative regulation of the noncanonical NF-kappa B pathway. J Biol Chem 282, 3688-94.

He, J.Q., Zarnegar, B., Oganesyan, G., Saha, S.K., Yamazaki, S., Doyle, S.E., Dempsey, P.W. and Cheng, G. (2006) Rescue of TRAF3-null mice by p100 NF-kappa B deficiency. J Exp Med 203, 2413-8.

Hebenstreit, D., Horejs-Hoeck, J. and Duschl, A. (2005) JAK/STAT-dependent gene regulation by cytokines. Drug News Perspect 18, 243-9.

Hoe, H.S. and Rebeck, G.W. (2008) Regulated proteolysis of APP and ApoE receptors. Mol Neurobiol 37, 64-72.

Hokama, Y., Empey-Campora, C., Hara, C., Higa, N., Siu, N., Lau, R., Kuribayashi, T. and Yabusaki, K. (2008) Acute phase phospholipids related to the cardiolipin of mitochondria in the sera of patients with chronic fatigue syndrome (CFS), chronic Ciguatera fish poisoning (CCFP), and other diseases attributed to chemicals, Gulf War, and marine toxins. J Clin Lab Anal 22, 99-105.

Howlin, J., Rosenkvist, J. and Andersson, T. (2008) TNK2 preserves epidermal growth factor receptor expression on the cell surface and enhances migration and invasion of human breast cancer cells. Breast Cancer Res 10, R36.

Huang, S., Pettaway, C.A., Uehara, H., Bucana, C.D. and Fidler, I.J. (2001) Blockade of NF-kappaB activity in human prostate cancer cells is associated with suppression of angiogenesis, invasion, and metastasis. Oncogene 20, 4188-97.

Huang, Z., Fasco, M.J., Figge, H.L., Keyomarsi, K. and Kaminsky, L.S. (1996) Expression of cytochromes P450 in human breast tissue and tumors. Drug Metab Dispos 24, 899-905.

Huber, A.R., Kunkel, S.L., Todd, R.F., 3rd and Weiss, S.J. (1991) Regulation of transendothelial neutrophil migration by endogenous interleukin-8. Science 254, 99-102.

Huh, M.I., Chang, Y. and Jung, J.C. (2009) Temporal and spatial distribution of TGF-beta isoforms and signaling intermediates in corneal regenerative wound repair. Histol Histopathol 24, 1405-16.

Hutvagner, G. and Zamore, P.D. (2002) A microRNA in a multiple-turnover RNAi enzyme complex. Science 297, 2056-60.

Ihle, J.N. (2001) The Stat family in cytokine signaling. Curr Opin Cell Biol 13, 211-7.

Inoue, A., Omoto, Y., Yamaguchi, Y., Kiyama, R. and Hayashi, S.I. (2004) Transcription factor EGR3 is involved in the estrogen-signaling pathway in breast cancer cells. Journal of molecular endocrinology 32, 649-61.

Ito, K., Hanazawa, T., Tomita, K., Barnes, P.J. and Adcock, I.M. (2004) Oxidative stress reduces histone deacetylase 2 activity and enhances IL-8 gene expression: role of tyrosine nitration. Biochem Biophys Res Commun 315, 240-5.

Itoh, S. and ten Dijke, P. (2007) Negative regulation of TGF-beta receptor/Smad signal transduction. Curr Opin Cell Biol 19, 176-84.

Jaeschke, A., Rincon, M., Doran, B., Reilly, J., Neuberg, D., Greiner, D.L., Shultz, L.D., Rossini, A.A., Flavell, R.A. and Davis, R.J. (2005) Disruption of the Jnk2 (Mapk9) gene reduces destructive insulitis and diabetes in a mouse model of type I diabetes. Proc Natl Acad Sci U S A 102, 6931-5.

Janssen, E.M., Droin, N.M., Lemmens, E.E., Pinkoski, M.J., Bensinger, S.J., Ehst, B.D., Griffith, T.S., Green, D.R. and Schoenberger, S.P. (2005) $CD4^+$ T-cell help controls $CD8^+$ T-cell memory via TRAIL-mediated activation-induced cell death. Nature 434, 88-93.

Jazin, E.E., Soderstrom, S., Ebendal, T. and Larhammar, D. (1997) Embryonic expression of the mRNA for the rat homologue of the fusin/CXCR-4 HIV-1 co-receptor. J Neuroimmunol 79, 148-54.

Jia, D., Rahbar, R., Chan, R.W., Lee, S.M., Chan, M.C., Wang, B.X., Baker, D.P., Sun, B., Peiris, J.S., Nicholls, J.M., Fish, E.N. (2010) Influenza virus non-structrual protein 1 (NS1) disrupt interferon signaling. PLoS One 5, e13927.

Jiang, H. and Wang, Y.C. (1996) [Cyclin-dependent kinase inhibitors in mammal cells]. Sheng Li Ke Xue Jin Zhan 27, 107-12.

Jiang, Y.M., Yamamoto, M., Kobayashi, Y., Yoshihara, T., Liang, Y., Terao, S., Takeuchi, H., Ishigaki, S., Katsuno, M., Adachi, H., Niwa, J., Tanaka, F., Doyu, M., Yoshida, M., Hashizume, Y. and Sobue, G. (2005) Gene expression profile of spinal motor neurons in sporadic amyotrophic lateral sclerosis. Annals of neurology 57, 236-51.

Jones, D.E., Hollingsworth, K.G., Taylor, R., Blamire, A.M. and Newton, J.L. (2009) Abnormalities in pH handling by peripheral muscle and potential regulation by the autonomic nervous system in chronic fatigue syndrome. J Intern Med 267, 394-401.

Ju, X., Zenke, M., Hart, D.N. and Clark, G.J. (2008) CD300a/c regulate type I interferon and TNF-alpha secretion by human plasmacytoid dendritic cells stimulated with TLR7 and TLR9 ligands. Blood 112, 1184-94.

Kagami, S., Nakajima, H., Suto, A., Hirose, K., Suzuki, K., Morita, S., Kato, I., Saito, Y., Kitamura, T. and Iwamoto, I. (2001) Stat5a regulates T helper cell differentiation by several distinct mechanisms. Blood 97, 2358-65.

Kajimoto, K., Shao, D., Takagi, H., Maceri, G., Zablocki, D., Mukai, H., Ono, Y. and Sadoshima, J. (2011) Hypotonic swelling-induced activation of PKN1 mediates cell survival in cardiac myocytes. American journal of physiology. Heart and circulatory physiology 300, H191-200.

Kamimura, D., Ishihara, K. and Hirano, T. (2003) IL-6 signal transduction and its physiological roles: the signal orchestration model. Rev Physiol Biochem Pharmacol 149, 1-38.

Karvonen, U., Janne, O.A. and Palvimo, J.J. (2006) Androgen receptor regulates nuclear trafficking and nuclear domain residency of corepressor HDAC7 in a ligand-dependent fashion. Exp Cell Res 312, 3165-83.

Kasler, H.G. and Verdin, E. (2007) Histone deacetylase 7 functions as a key regulator of genes involved in both positive and negative selection of thymocytes. Mol Cell Biol 27, 5184-200.

Kato, T., Jr., Gotoh, Y., Hoffmann, A. and Ono, Y. (2008) Negative regulation of constitutive NF-kappaB and JNK signaling by PKN1-mediated phosphorylation of TRAF1. Genes Cells 13, 509-20.

Kaushik, N., Fear, D., Richards, S.C., McDermott, C.R., Nuwaysir, E.F., Kellam, P., Harrison, T.J., Wilkinson, R.J., Tyrrell, D.A., Holgate, S.T. and Kerr, J.R. (2005) Gene expression in peripheral blood mononuclear cells from patients with chronic fatigue syndrome. J Clin Pathol 58, 826-32.

Kayagaki, N., Yamaguchi, N., Nakayama, M., Eto, H., Okumura, K. and Yagita, H. (1999) Type I interferons (IFNs) regulate tumor necrosis factor-related apoptosis-inducing ligand (TRAIL) expression on human T cells: A novel mechanism for the antitumor effects of type I IFNs. J Exp Med 189, 1451-60.

Kennedy, G., Spence, V., Underwood, C. and Belch, J.J. (2004) Increased neutrophil apoptosis in chronic fatigue syndrome. J Clin Pathol 57, 891-3.

Kerr, J.R. (2008) Gene profiling of patients with chronic fatigue syndrome/myalgic encephalomyelitis. Curr Rheumatol Rep 10, 482-91.

Kerr, J.R., Petty, R., Burke, B., Gough, J., Fear, D., Sinclair, L.I., Mattey, D.L., Richards, S.C., Montgomery, J., Baldwin, D.A., Kellam, P., Harrison, T.J., Griffin, G.E., Main, J., Enlander, D., Nutt, D.J. and Holgate, S.T. (2008) Gene expression subtypes in patients with chronic fatigue syndrome/myalgic encephalomyelitis. J Infect Dis 197, 1171-84.

Khvorova, A., Lescoute, A., Westhof, E. and Jayasena, S.D. (2003) Sequence elements outside the hammerhead ribozyme catalytic core enable intracellular activity. Nat Struct Biol 10, 708-12.

Kim, S.H., Serezani, C.H., Okunishi, K., Zaslona, Z., Aronoff, D.M. and Peters-Golden, M. (2011) Distinct protein kinase A anchoring proteins direct prostaglandin E2 modulation of Toll-like receptor signaling in alveolar macrophages. J Biol Chem 286, 8875-83.

Kitamura, H., Kanehira, K., Okita, K., Morimatsu, M. and Saito, M. (2000) MAIL, a novel nuclear I kappa B protein that potentiates LPS-induced IL-6 production. FEBS Lett 485, 53-6.

Kohlhaas, S., Garden, O.A., Scudamore, C., Turner, M., Okkenhaug, K. and Vigorito, E. (2009) Cutting edge: the Foxp3 target miR-155 contributes to the development of regulatory T cells. J Immunol 182, 2578-82.

Kristiansen, O.P. and Mandrup-Poulsen, T. (2005) Interleukin-6 and diabetes: the good, the bad, or the indifferent? Diabetes 54 Suppl 2, S114-24.

Kuratsune, H., Kondo, K., Ikuta, K., Yamanishi, K., Watanabe, Y. and Kitani, T. (2001) [Chronic fatigue syndrome (CFS)]. Nihon Naika Gakkai Zasshi 90, 2431-7.

Lacy, P. (2006) Mechanisms of degranulation in neutrophils. Allergy Asthma Clin Immunol 2, 98-108.

Lahmers, K.K., Hedges, J.F., Jutila, M.A., Deng, M., Abrahamsen, M.S. and Brown, W.C. (2006) Comparative gene expression by WC1^{+} gammadelta and CD4^{+} alphabeta T lymphocytes, which respond to Anaplasma marginale, demonstrates higher expression of chemokines and other myeloid cell-associated genes by WC1^{+} gammadelta T cells. Journal of leukocyte biology 80, 939-52.

Lange, G., DeLuca, J., Maldjian, J.A., Lee, H., Tiersky, L.A. and Natelson, B.H. (1999) Brain MRI abnormalities exist in a subset of patients with chronic fatigue syndrome. J Neurol Sci 171, 3-7.

Lee, K.M., Jeon, S.M. and Cho, H.J. (2009) Tumor necrosis factor receptor 1 induces interleukin-6 upregulation through NF-kappaB in a rat neuropathic pain model. Eur J Pain 13, 794-806.

Leong J.W. and Fehniger, T. (2010) Human NK SET to kill. Blood 24, 117-118.

R., Lee, Y., Ahn, C., Han, J., Choi, H., Kim, J., Yim, J., Lee, J., Provost, P., Radmark, O., Kim, S. and Kim, V.N. (2003) The nuclear RNase III Drosha initiates microRNA processing. Nature 425, 415-9.

Lee, Y., Jeon, K., Lee, J.T., Kim, S. and Kim, V.N. (2002) MicroRNA maturation: stepwise processing and subcellular localization. EMBO J 21, 4663-70.

Leung, L. and Cahill, C.M. (2010) TNF-alpha and neuropathic pain--a review. J Neuroinflammation 7, 27.

Li, Q.J., Chau, J., Ebert, P.J., Sylvester, G., Min, H., Liu, G., Braich, R., Manoharan, M., Soutschek, J., Skare, P., Klein, L.O., Davis, M.M. and Chen, C.Z. (2007) miR-181a is an intrinsic modulator of T cell sensitivity and selection. Cell 129, 147-61.

Li, W. and Ruan, K. (2009) MicroRNA detection by microarray. Analytical and bioanalytical chemistry 394, 1117-24.

Light, A.R., White, A.T., Hughen, R.W. and Light, K.C. (2009) Moderate Exercise Increases Expression for Sensory, Adrenergic, and Immune Genes in Chronic Fatigue Syndrome Patients But Not in Normal Subjects. J Pain.

Lim, L.P., Lau, N.C., Garrett-Engele, P., Grimson, A., Schelter, J.M., Castle, J., Bartel, D.P., Linsley, P.S. and Johnson, J.M. (2005) Microarray analysis shows that some microRNAs downregulate large numbers of target mRNAs. Nature 433, 769-73.

Lin, J.X. and Leonard, W.J. (2000) The role of Stat5a and Stat5b in signaling by IL-2 family cytokines. Oncogene 19, 2566-76.

Lindberg, F.P., Gresham, H.D., Schwarz, E. and Brown, E.J. (1993) Molecular cloning of integrin-associated protein: an immunoglobulin family member with multiple membrane-spanning domains implicated in alpha v beta 3-dependent ligand binding. J Cell Biol 123, 485-96.

Lingel, A., Simon, B., Izaurralde, E. and Sattler, M. (2003) Structure and nucleic-acid binding of the Drosophila Argonaute 2 PAZ domain. Nature 426, 465-9.

Lloyd, A.R., Hickie, I., Boughton, C.R., Spencer, O. and Wakefield, D. (1990) Prevalence of chronic fatigue syndrome in an Australian population. Med J Australia 153, 522-528.

Lu, J., Getz, G., Miska, E.A., Alvarez-Saavedra, E., Lamb, J., Peck, D., Sweet-Cordero, A., Ebert, B.L., Mak, R.H., Ferrando, A.A., Downing, J.R., Jacks, T., Horvitz, H.R. and Golub, T.R. (2005) MicroRNA expression profiles classify human cancers. Nature 435, 834-8.

Lu, L.F., Thai, T.H., Calado, D.P., Chaudhry, A., Kubo, M., Tanaka, K., Loeb, G.B., Lee, H., Yoshimura, A., Rajewsky, K. and Rudensky, A.Y. (2009) Foxp3-dependent microRNA155 confers competitive fitness to regulatory T cells by targeting SOCS1 protein. Immunity 30, 80-91.

Lu, Y.C., Yeh, W.C. and Ohashi, P.S. (2008) LPS/TLR4 signal transduction pathway. Cytokine 42, 145-51.

Madueno, J.A., Munoz, E., Blazquez, V., Gonzalez, R., Aparicio, P. and Pena, J. (1993) The CD26 antigen is coupled to protein tyrosine phosphorylation and implicated in CD16-mediated lysis in natural killer cells. Scandinavian journal of immunology 37, 425-9.

Maher, K.J., Klimas, N.G. and Fletcher, M.A. (2005) Chronic fatigue syndrome is associated with diminished intracellular perforin. Clinical and experimental immunology 142, 505-11.

Marie, J.C., Letterio, J.J., Gavin, M. and Rudensky, A.Y. (2005) TGF-beta1 maintains suppressor function and Foxp3 expression in $CD4^+CD25^+$ regulatory T cells. J Exp Med 201, 1061-7.

Marson, A., Kretschmer, K., Frampton, G.M., Jacobsen, E.S., Polansky, J.K., MacIsaac, K.D., Levine, S.S., Fraenkel, E., von Boehmer, H. and Young, R.A. (2007) Foxp3 occupancy and regulation of key target genes during T-cell stimulation. Nature 445, 931-5.

Matsuoka, M. and Jeang, K.T. (2005) Human T-cell leukemia virus type I at age 25: a progress report. Cancer Res 65, 4467-70.

McGeachy, M.J. and Cua, D.J. (2007) T cells doing it for themselves: TGF-beta regulation of Th1 and Th17 cells. Immunity 26, 547-9.

McGuire, M.J., Lipsky, P.E. and Thiele, D.L. (1997) Cloning and characterization of the cDNA encoding mouse dipeptidyl peptidase I (cathepsin C). Biochim Biophys Acta 1351, 267-73.

Meyer-Lindenberg, A., Kohn, P.D., Kolachana, B., Kippenhan, S., McInerney-Leo, A., Nussbaum, R., Weinberger, D.R. and Berman, K.F. (2005) Midbrain dopamine and prefrontal function in humans: interaction and modulation by COMT genotype. Nat Neurosci 8, 594-6.

Miller, C., Wang, L., Ostergaard, E., Dan, P. and Saada, A. (2011) The interplay between SUCLA2, SUCLG2, and mitochondrial DNA depletion. Biochim Biophys Acta 1812, 625-9.

Mishima, Y., Giraldez, A.J., Takeda, Y., Fujiwara, T., Sakamoto, H., Schier, A.F. and Inoue, K. (2006) Differential regulation of germline mRNAs in soma and germ cells by zebrafish miR-430. Curr Biol 16, 2135-42.

Moepps, B., Frodl, R., Rodewald, H.R., Baggiolini, M. and Gierschik, P. (1997) Two murine homologues of the human chemokine receptor CXCR4 mediating stromal cell-derived factor 1alpha activation of Gi2 are differentially expressed in vivo. Eur J Immunol 27, 2102-12.

Moore, K.W., de Waal Malefyt, R., Coffman, R.L. and O'Garra, A. (2001) Interleukin-10 and the interleukin-10 receptor. Annu Rev Immunol 19, 683-765.

Morin, R.D., O'Connor, M.D., Griffith, M., Kuchenbauer, F., Delaney, A., Prabhu, A.L., Zhao, Y., McDonald, H., Zeng, T., Hirst, M., Eaves, C.J. and Marra, M.A. (2008) Application of massively parallel sequencing to microRNA profiling and discovery in human embryonic stem cells. Genome research 18, 610-21.

Moriuchi, M., Moriuchi, H., Turner, W. and Fauci, A.S. (1998) Exposure to bacterial products renders macrophages highly susceptible to T-tropic HIV-1. J Clin Invest 102, 1540-50.

Morrison, G., Kilanowski, F., Davidson, D. and Dorin, J. (2002) Characterization of the mouse beta defensin 1, Defb1, mutant mouse model. Infect Immun 70, 3053-60.

Moser, C., Weiner, D.J., Lysenko, E., Bals, R., Weiser, J.N. and Wilson, J.M. (2002) beta-Defensin 1 contributes to pulmonary innate immunity in mice. Infect Immun 70, 3068-72.

Mourelatos, Z., Dostie, J., Paushkin, S., Sharma, A., Charroux, B., Abel, L., Rappsilber, J., Mann, M. and Dreyfuss, G. (2002) miRNPs: a novel class of ribonucleoproteins containing numerous microRNAs. Genes Dev 16, 720-8.

Mukaida, N. (2003) Pathophysiological roles of interleukin-8/CXCL8 in pulmonary diseases. Am J Physiol Lung Cell Mol Physiol 284, L566-77.

Myhill, S., Booth, N.E. and McLaren-Howard, J. (2009) Chronic fatigue syndrome and mitochondrial dysfunction. Int J Clin Exp Med 2, 1-16.

Newton, J.L., Okonkwo, O., Sutcliffe, K., Seth, A., Shin, J. and Jones, D.E. (2007) Symptoms of autonomic dysfunction in chronic fatigue syndrome. QJM 100, 519-26.

Nizet, V. and Johnson, R.S. (2009) Interdependence of hypoxic and innate immune responses. Nat Rev Immunol 9, 609-17.

Nowlan, M.L., Drewe, E., Bulsara, H., Esposito, N., Robins, R.A., Tighe, P.J., Powell, R.J. and Todd, I. (2006) Systemic cytokine levels and the effects of etanercept in TNF receptor-associated periodic syndrome (TRAPS) involving a C33Y mutation in TNFRSF1A. Rheumatology (Oxford) 45, 31-7.

Nozell, S., Laver, T., Patel, K. and Benveniste, E.N. (2006) Mechanism of IFN-beta-mediated inhibition of IL-8 gene expression in astroglioma cells. J Immunol 177, 822-30.

O'Connell, R.M., Taganov, K.D., Boldin, M.P., Cheng, G. and Baltimore, D. (2007) MicroRNA-155 is induced during the macrophage inflammatory response. Proc Natl Acad Sci U S A 104, 1604-9.

O'Shea, J.J., Gadina, M. and Schreiber, R.D. (2002) Cytokine signaling in 2002: new surprises in the Jak/Stat pathway. Cell 109 Suppl, S121-31.

Oberle, N., Eberhardt, N., Falk, C.S., Krammer, P.H. and Suri-Payer, E. (2007) Rapid suppression of cytokine transcription in human $CD4^{+}CD25$ T cells by $CD4^{+}Foxp3^{+}$ regulatory T cells: independence of IL-2 consumption, TGF-beta, and various inhibitors of TCR signaling. J Immunol 179, 3578-87.

Orlinick, J.R. and Chao, M.V. (1998) TNF-related ligands and their receptors. Cell Signal 10, 543-51.

Panousis, C.G., Evans, G. and Zuckerman, S.H. (2001) TGF-beta increases cholesterol efflux and ABC-1 expression in macrophage-derived foam cells: opposing the effects of IFN-gamma. J Lipid Res 42, 856-63.

Park, J.H. and Levitt, L. (1993) Overexpression of mitogen-activated protein kinase (ERK1) enhances T-cell cytokine gene expression: role of AP1, NF-AT, and NF-KB. Blood 82, 2470-7.

Parkos, C.A., Colgan, S.P., Liang, T.W., Nusrat, A., Bacarra, A.E., Carnes, D.K. and Madara, J.L. (1996) CD47 mediates post-adhesive events required for neutrophil migration across polarized intestinal epithelia. J Cell Biol 132, 437-50.

Pasi, A., Bozzini, S., Carlo-Stella, N., Martinetti, M., Bombardieri, S., De Silvestri, A., Salvaneschi, L. and Cuccia, M. (2011) Excess of activating killer cell immunoglobulinlike receptors and lack of HLA-Bw4 ligands: a twoedged weapon in chronic fatigue syndrome. Molecular medicine reports 4, 535-40.

Pham, C.T. and Ley, T.J. (1999) Dipeptidyl peptidase I is required for the processing and activation of granzymes A and B in vivo. Proc Natl Acad Sci U S A 96, 8627-32.

Pickering, M., Cumiskey, D. and O'Connor, J.J. (2005) Actions of TNF-alpha on glutamatergic synaptic transmission in the central nervous system. Exp Physiol 90, 663-70.

Pierce, K.L., Premont, R.T. and Lefkowitz, R.J. (2002) Seven-transmembrane receptors. Nat Rev Mol Cell Biol 3, 639-50.

Plioplys, A.V. and Plioplys, S. (1995) Electron-microscopic investigation of muscle mitochondria in chronic fatigue syndrome. Neuropsychobiology 32, 175-81.

Pollard, T.D. (2007) Regulation of actin filament assembly by Arp2/3 complex and formins. Annu Rev Biophys Biomol Struct 36, 451-77.

Pradelli, L.A., Beneatea, M., Ricci, J.E. (2010) Mitchondrialcontrol of caspases-dependent and -independent cell death.Cell Mol Life Sci 67, 15898

Presson, A.P., Sobel, E.M., Papp, J.C., Suarez, C.J., Whistler, T., Rajeevan, M.S., Vernon, S.D. and Horvath, S. (2008) Integrated weighted gene co-expression network analysis with an application to chronic fatigue syndrome. BMC Syst Biol 2, 95.

Rajeevan, M.S., Smith, A.K., Dimulescu, I., Unger, E.R., Vernon, S.D., Heim, C. and Reeves, W.C. (2007) Glucocorticoid receptor polymorphisms and haplotypes associated with chronic fatigue syndrome. Genes Brain Behav 6, 167-76.

Rameil, P., Lecine, P., Ghysdael, J., Gouilleux, F., Kahn-Perles, B. and Imbert, J. (2000) IL-2 and long-term T cell activation induce physical and functional interaction between STAT5 and ETS transcription factors in human T cells. Oncogene 19, 2086-97.

Rao, A., Luo, C. and Hogan, P.G. (1997a) Transcription factors of the NFAT family: regulation and function. Annu Rev Immunol 15, 707-47.

Rao, N.V., Rao, G.V. and Hoidal, J.R. (1997b) Human dipeptidyl-peptidase I. Gene characterization, localization, and expression. J Biol Chem 272, 10260-5.

Reynolds, C.A., Hong, M.G., Eriksson, U.K., Blennow, K., Johansson, B., Malmberg, B., Berg, S., Gatz, M., Pedersen, N.L., Bennet, A.M. and Prince, J.A. (2010) Sequence variation in SORL1 and dementia risk in Swedes. Neurogenetics 11, 139-42.

Reynolds, G.P., Templeman, L.A. and Godlewska, B.R. (2006) Pharmacogenetics of schizophrenia. Expert opinion on pharmacotherapy 7, 1429-40.

Rodriguez, A., Vigorito, E., Clare, S., Warren, M.V., Couttet, P., Soond, D.R., van Dongen, S., Grocock, R.J., Das, P.P., Miska, E.A., Vetrie, D., Okkenhaug, K., Enright, A.J., Dougan, G., Turner, M. and Bradley, A. (2007) Requirement of bic/microRNA-155 for normal immune function. Science 316, 608-11.

Rorbach, J., Richter, R., Wessels, H.J., Wydro, M., Pekalski, M., Farhoud, M., Kuhl, I., Gaisne, M., Bonnefoy, N., Smeitink, J.A., Lightowlers, R.N. and Chrzanowska-Lightowlers, Z.M. (2008) The human mitochondrial ribosome recycling factor is essential for cell viability. Nucleic Acids Res 36, 5787-99.

Russell, L. and Garrett-Sinha, L.A. (2010) Transcription factor Ets-1 in cytokine and chemokine gene regulation. Cytokine 51, 217-26.

Safford, M., Collins, S., Lutz, M.A., Allen, A., Huang, C.T., Kowalski, J., Blackford, A., Horton, M.R., Drake, C., Schwartz, R.H. and Powell, J.D. (2005) Egr-2 and Egr-3 are negative regulators of T cell activation. Nat Immunol 6, 472-80.

Saiki, T., Kawai, T., Morita, K., Ohta, M., Saito, T., Rokutan, K. and Ban, N. (2008) Identification of marker genes for differential diagnosis of chronic fatigue syndrome. Mol Med 14, 599-607.

Salaun, B., Yamamoto, T., Badran, B., Tsunetsugu-Yokota, Y., Roux, A., Baitsch, L., Rouas, R., Fayyad-Kazan, H., Baumgaertner, P., Devevre, E., Ramesh, A., Braun, M., Speiser, D., Autran, B., Martiat, P., Appay, V. and Romero, P. (2011) Differentiation associated regulation of microRNA expression in vivo in human $CD8^+$ T cell subsets. Journal of translational medicine 9, 44.

Sanchez-Capelo, A. (2005) Dual role for TGF-beta1 in apoptosis. Cytokine Growth Factor Rev 16, 15-34.

Schaefer, U., Voloshanenko, O., Willen, D. and Walczak, H. (2007) TRAIL: a multifunctional cytokine. Front Biosci 12, 3813-24.

Schindler, C. (1999) Cytokines and JAK-STAT signaling. Exp Cell Res 253, 7-14.

Schindler, C., Levy, D.E. and Decker, T. (2007) JAK-STAT signaling: from interferons to cytokines. J Biol Chem 282, 20059-63.

Schutzer, S.E., Angel, T.E., Liu, T., Schepmoes, A.A., Clauss, T.R., Adkins, J.N., Camp, D.G., Holland, B.K., Bergquist, J., Coyle, P.K., Smith, R.D., Fallon, B.A. and Natelson, B.H. (2011a) Distinct cerebrospinal fluid proteomes differentiate post-treatment lyme disease from chronic fatigue syndrome. PLoS One 6, e17287.

Schutzer, S.E., Rounds, M.A., Natelson, B.H., Ecker, D.J. and Eshoo, M.W. (2011b) Analysis of cerebrospinal fluid from chronic fatigue syndrome patients for multiple human ubiquitous viruses and xenotropic murine leukemia-related virus. Ann Neurol 69, 735-8.

Schwartz, R.B., Garada, B.M., Komaroff, A.L., Tice, H.M., Gleit, M., Jolesz, F.A. and Holman, B.L. (1994) Detection of intracranial abnormalities in patients with chronic fatigue syndrome: comparison of MR imaging and SPECT. AJR Am J Roentgenol 162, 935-41.

Scott, J.D. (1991) Cyclic nucleotide-dependent protein kinases. Pharmacol Ther 50, 123-45.

See, D.M., Cimoch, P., Chou, S., Chang, J. and Tilles, J. (1998) The in vitro immunomodulatory effects of glyconutrients on peripheral blood mononuclear cells of patients with chronic fatigue syndrome. Integr Physiol Behav Sci 33, 280-7.

Sen, G.C. (2001) Viruses and interferons. Annu Rev Microbiol 55, 255-81.

Sha, W.C., Liou, H.C., Tuomanen, E.I. and Baltimore, D. (1995) Targeted disruption of the p50 subunit of NF-kappa B leads to multifocal defects in immune responses. Cell 80, 321-30.

Sharpe, M.C., Archard, L.C., Bantanatvala, J.E., Borysiewicz, L.K., Clare, A.W., David, A., Edwards, R.H., Hawton, K.E., Lambert, H.P., Lane, R.J. & et al. (1991) A report--chronic fatigue syndrome: guidelines for research. J R Soc Med, 84, 118-21.

Shen, Y.L., Jiang, Y.G., Greenlee, A.R., Zhou, L.L. and Liu, L.H. (2009) MicroRNA expression profiles and miR-10a target in anti-benzo[a] pyrene-7, 8-diol-9, 10-epoxide-transformed human 16HBE cells. Biomed Environ Sci 22, 14-21.

Shevach, E.M. (2010) TGF-Beta to the rescue. Immunity 32, 585-7.

Shibata, N., Ohnuma, T., Baba, H., Higashi, S., Nishioka, K. and Arai, H. (2008) Genetic association between SORL1 polymorphisms and Alzheimer's disease in a Japanese population. Dement Geriatr Cogn Disord 26, 161-4.

Shimada, T., Hayes, C.L., Yamazaki, H., Amin, S., Hecht, S.S., Guengerich, F.P. and Sutter, T.R. (1996) Activation of chemically diverse procarcinogens by human cytochrome P-450 1B1. Cancer Res 56, 2979-84.

Skowera, A., Cleare, A., Blair, D., Bevis, L., Wessely, S.C. and Peakman, M. (2004) High levels of type 2 cytokine-producing cells in chronic fatigue syndrome. Clin Exp Immunol 135, 294-302.

Sparkman, L. and Boggaram, V. (2004) Nitric oxide increases IL-8 gene transcription and mRNA stability to enhance IL-8 gene expression in lung epithelial cells. Am J Physiol Lung Cell Mol Physiol 287, L764-73.

Strobl, H. and Knapp, W. (1999) TGF-beta1 regulation of dendritic cells. Microbes Infect 1, 1283-90.

Studer, M., Gavalas, A., Marshall, H., Ariza-McNaughton, L., Rijli, F.M., Chambon, P. and Krumlauf, R. (1998) Genetic interactions between Hoxa1 and Hoxb1 reveal new roles in regulation of early hindbrain patterning. Development 125, 1025-36.

Su, D.M., Navarre, S., Oh, W.J., Condie, B.G. and Manley, N.R. (2003) A domain of Foxn1 required for crosstalk-dependent thymic epithelial cell differentiation. Nat Immunol 4, 1128-35.

Sun, L., Finnegan, C.M., Kish-Catalone, T., Blumenthal, R., Garzino-Demo, P., La Terra Maggiore, G.M., Berrone, S., Kleinman, C., Wu, Z., Abdelwahab, S., Lu, W. and Garzino-Demo, A. (2005) Human beta-defensins suppress human immunodeficiency virus infection: potential role in mucosal protection. J Virol 79, 14318-29.

Sun, W., Julie Li, Y.S., Huang, H.D., Shyy, J.Y. and Chien, S. (2010) microRNA: a master regulator of cellular processes for bioengineering systems. Annual review of biomedical engineering 12, 1-27.

Taganov, K.D., Boldin, M.P., Chang, K.J. and Baltimore, D. (2006) NF-kappaB-dependent induction of microRNA miR-146, an inhibitor targeted to signaling proteins of innate immune responses. Proc Natl Acad Sci U S A 103, 12481-6.

Tasken, K., Skalhegg, B.S., Tasken, K.A., Solberg, R., Knutsen, H.K., Levy, F.O., Sandberg, M., Orstavik, S., Larsen, T., Johansen, A.K., Vang, T., Schrader, H.P., Reinton, N.T., Torgersen, K.M., Hansson, V. and Jahnsen, T. (1997) Structure, function, and regulation of human cAMP-dependent protein kinases. Adv Second Messenger Phosphoprotein Res 31, 191-204.

Thai, T.H., Calado, D.P., Casola, S., Ansel, K.M., Xiao, C., Xue, Y., Murphy, A., Frendewey, D., Valenzuela, D., Kutok, J.L., Schmidt-Supprian, M., Rajewsky, N., Yancopoulos, G., Rao, A. and Rajewsky, K. (2007) Regulation of the germinal center response by microRNA-155. Science 316, 604-8.

Ter Wolbeek, M., van Doornen, L.J.P., Kavelaars, A. And Heijnen, C.J. (2008) Predictors of persistent and new-onset of fatigue in adolescent girls. Pediatrics 121, e449.

Thomas, R.S., Tymms, M.J., McKinlay, L.H., Shannon, M.F., Seth, A. and Kola, I. (1997) ETS1, NFkappaB and AP1 synergistically transactivate the human GM-CSF promoter. Oncogene 14, 2845-55.

Ticchioni, M., Deckert, M., Mary, F., Bernard, G., Brown, E.J. and Bernard, A. (1997) Integrin-associated protein (CD47) is a comitogenic molecule on CD3-activated human T cells. J Immunol 158, 677-84.

Tili, E., Michaille, J.J., Cimino, A., Costinean, S., Dumitru, C.D., Adair, B., Fabbri, M., Alder, H., Liu, C.G., Calin, G.A. and Croce, C.M. (2007) Modulation of miR-155 and miR-125b levels following lipopolysaccharide/TNF-alpha stimulation and their possible roles in regulating the response to endotoxin shock. J Immunol 179, 5082-9.

Turnbull, I.R. and Colonna, M. (2007) Activating and inhibitory functions of DAP12. Nat Rev Immunol 7, 155-61.

Ursini, F., Succurro, E., Grembiale, A., Gagliardi, D.A. and Arturi, F. (2010) [The HPA axis in the pathogenesis of chronic fatigue syndrome]. La Clinica terapeutica 161, 461-4.

Vernon, S.D., Unger, E.R., Dimulescu, I.M., Rajeevan, M. and Reeves, W.C. (2002) Utility of the blood for gene expression profiling and biomarker discovery in chronic fatigue syndrome. Disease markers 18, 193-9.

Vita, N., Lefort, S., Sozzani, P., Reeb, R., Richards, S., Borysiewicz, L.K., Ferrara, P. and Labeta, M.O. (1997) Detection and biochemical characteristics of the receptor for complexes of soluble CD14 and bacterial lipopolysaccharide. J Immunol 158, 3457-62.

Vojdani, A., Mordechai, E. and Brautbar, N. (1997) Abnormal apoptosis and cell cycle progression in humans exposed to methyl tertiary-butyl ether and benzene contaminating water. Hum Exp Toxicol 16, 485-94.

Waclavicek, M., Majdic, O., Stulnig, T., Berger, M., Baumruker, T., Knapp, W. and Pickl, W.F. (1997) T cell stimulation via CD47: agonistic and antagonistic effects of CD47 monoclonal antibody 1/1A4. J Immunol 159, 5345-54.

Wahl, S.M., Swisher, J., McCartney-Francis, N. and Chen, W. (2004) TGF-beta: the perpetrator of immune suppression by regulatory T cells and suicidal T cells. J Leukoc Biol 76, 15-24.

Wahl, S.M., Wen, J. and Moutsopoulos, N. (2006) TGF-beta: a mobile purveyor of immune privilege. Immunol Rev 213, 213-27.

Walsh, C.M., Zainal, N.Z., Middleton, S.J. and Paykel, E.S. (2001) A family history study of chronic fatigue syndrome. Psychiatric genetics 11, 123-8.

Wang, M.J., Zhou, Z.G., Wang, L., Li, Y., Zhang, P., Zhang, Y., Cui, C.F. and Zhou, B. (2009a) [Genotyping of AKAP10 gene 2073A/G single nucleotide polymorphism by TaqMan probe real-time PCR]. Sichuan Da Xue Xue Bao Yi Xue Ban 40, 275-8.

Wang, M.J., Zhou, Z.G., Wang, L., Yu, Y.Y., Zhang, P., Zhang, Y., Cui, C.F., Yang, L., Li, Y., Zhou, B. and Sun, X.F. (2009b) The Ile646Val (2073A>G) polymorphism in the kinase-binding domain of A-kinase anchoring protein 10 and the risk of colorectal cancer. Oncology 76, 199-204.

Wang, S.E., Wu, F.Y., Shin, I., Qu, S. and Arteaga, C.L. (2005) Transforming growth factor (TGF-)-Smad target gene protein tyrosine phosphatase receptor type kappa is required for TGF- function. Mol Cell Biol 25, 4703-15.

Wang, X., Chen, Y., Ren, J. and Qu, X. (2011) Small interfering RNA for effective cancer therapies. Mini reviews in medicinal chemistry 11, 114-24.

Wang, D., John, S.A., Clements, J.L., Percy, D.H., Barton, K.P., Garrett-Sinha, L.A. (2005) Ets-1 deficiency leads to altered B cell differentiation, hyperresponsiveness to TLR9 and autoimmune disease. Int Immunol 17, 1179-1191.

Washbourne, P., Thompson, P.M., Carta, M., Costa, E.T., Mathews, J.R., Lopez-Bendito, G., Molnar, Z., Becher, M.W., Valenzuela, C.F., Partridge, L.D. and Wilson, M.C. (2002) Genetic ablation of the t-SNARE SNAP-25 distinguishes mechanisms of neuroexocytosis. Nat Neurosci 5, 19-26.

Wasylyk, B., Hagman, J. and Gutierrez-Hartmann, A. (1998) Ets transcription factors: nuclear effectors of the Ras-MAP-kinase signaling pathway. Trends Biochem Sci 23, 213-6.

Wehkamp, J., Salzman, N.H., Porter, E., Nuding, S., Weichenthal, M., Petras, R.E., Shen, B., Schaeffeler, E., Schwab, M., Linzmeier, R., Feathers, R.W., Chu, H., Lima, H., Jr., Fellermann, K., Ganz, T., Stange, E.F. and Bevins, C.L. (2005) Reduced Paneth cell alpha-defensins in ileal Crohn's disease. Proc Natl Acad Sci U S A 102, 18129-34.

Whistler, T., Jones, J.F., Unger, E.R. and Vernon, S.D. (2005) Exercise responsive genes measured in peripheral blood of women with chronic fatigue syndrome and matched control subjects. BMC Physiol 5, 5.

Whistler, T., Unger, E.R., Nisenbaum, R. and Vernon, S.D. (2003) Integration of gene expression, clinical, and epidemiologic data to characterize Chronic Fatigue Syndrome. J Transl Med 1, 10.

Wright, S.D., Ramos, R.A., Tobias, P.S., Ulevitch, R.J. and Mathison, J.C. (1990) CD14, a receptor for complexes of lipopolysaccharide (LPS) and LPS binding protein. Science 249, 1431-3.

Wu, H., Neilson, J.R., Kumar, P., Manocha, M., Shankar, P., Sharp, P.A. and Manjunath, N. (2007) miRNA Profiling of Naı¨ve, Effector and Memory CD8 T Cells. PLoS One 2, e1020.

Wu, L., Fan, J. and Belasco, J.G. (2006) MicroRNAs direct rapid deadenylation of mRNA. Proc Natl Acad Sci U S A 103, 4034-9.

Wyrwicz, L.S., Gaj, P., Hoffmann, M., Rychlewski, L. and Ostrowski, J. (2007) A common cis-element in promoters of protein synthesis and cell cycle genes. Acta Biochim Pol 54, 89-98.

Xie, K. (2001) Interleukin-8 and human cancer biology. Cytokine Growth Factor Rev 12, 375-91.

Xu, B., Doughman, Y., Turakhia, M., Jiang, W., Landsettle, C.E., Agani, F.H., Semenza, G.L., Watanabe, M. and Yang, Y.C. (2007) Partial rescue of defects in Cited2-deficient embryos by HIF-1alpha heterozygosity. Dev Biol 301, 130-40.

Yamazaki, S., Muta, T. and Takeshige, K. (2001) A novel IkappaB protein, IkappaB-zeta, induced by proinflammatory stimuli, negatively regulates nuclear factor-kappaB in the nuclei. J Biol Chem 276, 27657-62.

Yang, D., Chertov, O., Bykovskaia, S.N., Chen, Q., Buffo, M.J., Shogan, J., Anderson, M., Schroder, J.M., Wang, J.M., Howard, O.M. and Oppenheim, J.J. (1999) Beta-defensins: linking innate and adaptive immunity through dendritic and T cell CCR6. Science 286, 525-8.

Yang, L., Cohn, L., Zhang, D.H., Homer, R., Ray, A. and Ray, P. (1998) Essential role of nuclear factor kappaB in the induction of eosinophilia in allergic airway inflammation. J Exp Med 188, 1739-50.

Yoshimura, A., Wakabayashi, Y. and Mori, T. (2010) Cellular and molecular basis for the regulation of inflammation by TGF-beta. J Biochem 147, 781-92.

Yu, D., Tan, A.H., Hu, X., Athanasopoulos, V., Simpson, N., Silva, D.G., Hutloff, A., Giles, K.M., Leedman, P.J., Lam, K.P., Goodnow, C.C. and Vinuesa, C.G. (2007) Roquin represses autoimmunity by limiting inducible T-cell co-stimulator messenger RNA. Nature 450, 299-303.

Yu, E.Z., Li, Y.Y., Liu, X.H., Kagan, E. and McCarron, R.M. (2004) Antiapoptotic action of hypoxia-inducible factor-1 alpha in human endothelial cells. Lab Invest 84, 553-61.

Yuan, X., Naguib, S. and Wu, Z. (2011) Recent advances of siRNA delivery by nanoparticles. Expert opinion on drug delivery 8, 521-36.

Zetterberg, H., Blennow, K. and Hanse, E. (2010) Amyloid beta and APP as biomarkers for Alzheimer's disease. Exp Gerontol 45, 23-9.

Zhang, C. and Wong-Riley, M.T. (2000) Depolarizing stimulation upregulates GA-binding protein in neurons: a transcription factor involved in the bigenomic expression of cytochrome oxidase subunits. Eur J Neurosci 12, 1013-23.

Zhang, J.Z., Sinha, M., Luxon, B.A. and Yu, X.J. (2004) Survival strategy of obligately intracellular Ehrlichia chaffeensis: novel modulation of immune response and host cell cycles. Infect Immun 72, 498-507.

Zhang, X., Jin, J., Peng, X., Ramgolam, V.S. and Markovic-Plese, S. (2008) Simvastatin inhibits IL-17 secretion by targeting multiple IL-17-regulatory cytokines and by inhibiting the expression of IL-17 transcription factor RORC in $CD4^+$ lymphocytes. J Immunol 180, 6988-96.

Zhang, X.R., Zhang, L.Y., Devadas, S., Li, L., Keegan, A.D. and Shi, Y.F. (2003) Reciprocal expression of TRAIL and CD95L in Th1 and Th2 cells: role of apoptosis in T helper subset differentiation. Cell Death Differ 10, 203-10.

Zhang, Y., Zhang, J., Tian, C., Xiao, Y., He, C., Li, X., Boqati, A., Huang, J., Fan, H. (2010) The -308 G/A polymorphism in TNF-α gene is associated with asthma risk: an update by meta analysis. J Clin Immunol 31, 174-85.

Zhao, L., Furebring, M., Xu, S. and Venge, P. (2004) Subcellular localization and mobilization of carcinoembryonic antigen-related cell adhesion molecule 8 in human neutrophils. Br J Haematol 125, 666-73.

Zheng, Y., Josefowicz, S.Z., Kas, A., Chu, T.T., Gavin, M.A. and Rudensky, A.Y. (2007) Genome-wide analysis of Foxp3 target genes in developing and mature regulatory T cells. Nature 445, 936-40.

Zhou, S., Ou, R., Huang, L. and Moskophidis, D. (2002) Critical role for perforin-, Fas/FasL-, and TNFR1-mediated cytotoxic pathways in down-regulation of antigen-specific T cells during persistent viral infection. J Virol 76, 829-40.

Zou, Y.R., Kottmann, A.H., Kuroda, M., Taniuchi, I. and Littman, D.R. (1998) Function of the chemokine receptor CXCR4 in haematopoiesis and in cerebellar development. Nature 393, 595-9.

Zylbersztejn, K. and Galli, T. (2011) Vesicular traffic in cell navigation. FEBS J.

3

Integrated Analysis of Gene Expression and Genotype Variation Data for Chronic Fatigue Syndrome

Jungsoo Gim[1] and Taesung Park[1,2]
[1]*Intediscplinary program for bioinformatics, Seoul National University,*
[2]*Department of statistics, Seoul National University,*
South Korea

1. Introduction

In the past few years, high throughput technologies, such as gene expression microarrays and genotyping techniques, have provided efficient ways to measure gene expression levels and genotype variation on a genome-wide scale [Schena *et al.*, 1995; Howell *et al.*, 1999]. Various approaches have been proposed to analyse gene expression data and genotype variation data, in order to discover the complex network of biochemical processes of complex diseases such as chronic fatigue syndrome (CFS) [Presson *et al.*, 2008]. In the analysis of gene expression data, for example, the identification of differentially expressed genes between two groups has been of great interest, and various statistical tests have been conducted [Ghazalpour *et al.*, 2008; Brem *et al.*, 2002; Kang *et al.*, 2008]. In analysing genotype variation data, logistic regression has been commonly used to model the relationship between binary clinical outcomes and discrete predictors, such as genotypes [Henshall & Goddard, 1999; Coffey *et al.*, 2004].

Despite the availability of different levels of genome-wide data, most studies have been based on a separate analysis of single-level data to unravel complex biological mechanisms of CFS. Complex diseases such as CFS can be explained at different levels of biological mechanisms, including DNA, gene expression and phenotype levels. While there is a separate mechanism at each level, the mechanisms at different levels are closely related to each other in initiating and influencing CFS. Furthermore, CFS is expected to have complex etiology, which involves the action of many genes in addition to dynamic gene-environment interactions [Lin *et al.*, 2009]. Therefore, separate analyses of single-level data have a limitation in identifying and characterizing genes that are associated with the susceptibility of CFS. The integration of the different types of data (for example, gene expression, genotype variation and clinical outcomes) can provide more comprehensive information related to CFS, hence elucidate complex networks of gene interactions underlying CFS.

In this chapter, we provide an overview of the integrated statistical model (ISM) in order to characterize CFS, which involves integrating genotype variation data and gene expression data. The ISM elucidates the causal relationship between genetic variation, gene expression level and disease. The ISM consists of two steps. The first step is to determine the causal relationship. Based on the causal relationship determined at the first step, the second step identifies significant gene expression traits of which the effects on disease status or the responses to disease status are modified by the specific genotype variation. By applying the ISM procedure to a CFS dataset, we identified a list of potential causal genes for CFS, and found an evidence for a difference in genetic mechanisms of the etiology between CFS patient and control groups.

Our ISM analyses considering the different levels of data simultaneously, allowed us to elucidate disease susceptibility and differentially expressed genes of genetically different individuals. Some results even showed that integrating genotype and expression data may help the search for new directions for the treatment of CFS that are not being detected by using only one type of data. The integrated analysis provided more information than the two separate analyses of gene expression data and genotype variation data for characterizing CFS that has several possible causes.

2. An overview of Integrated Statistical Model (ISM)

2.1 From genotype to phenotype

In the era of the genome project, the belief came with was that we would answer the questions on how the genes function and how they are related to diseases. The genome project successfully sequenced DNA of various species, including the human. Not only sequencing the genomes, many studies have also identified the gene functions by modifying individual genes in several animals and plants. However, many questions remain unanswered. We still do not know the functions of numerous genes, whether thay are annotated or un-annotated. Especially predicting what genes are associated with disease-related phenotypic variants is of particular interest and still in vague. The problem is complicated, because

i. most phenotypes of medical interest are **complex diseases**, *i.e.*, more than one gene or environmental effect contributes to the phenotype occurrence,
ii. the underlying **molecular mechanism** regulating cellular functions **is complicated,** and
iii. **little genotypic data** (or information) of disease-related phenotypes is available.

High throughput technologies advance for acquiring genome-wide genotyping data of many individuals with and without disease phenotypes. It is of a particular interest to segregate genotypic difference between disease-affected individuals and controls. The variation of genotypes comes from additive and epistatic effects of alleles across multiple genes, resulting in many individuals with phenotypes. Some combinations of genotypic variants result in enhanced traits, whereas other combinations are deleterious to fitness in specific environments. Phenotypic alterations are usually in matters of amount, rather than in the presence or absence of a trait. The field of statistical genetics has developed various methods and tools to map such quantitative traits to regions of chromosomes. These chromosomal regions are known as quantitative trait loci (hereafter QTLs) and are described in terms of the percentage of the variation of a trait that can be attributed to each region.

2.1.1 Quantitative Trait Locus (QTL)

Quantitative traits refer to the characteristics or phenotypes that are quantitative, *i.e.*, vary in degree or continuously, such as height, while dichotomous or discrete traits have two or several characteristic values. A QTL is a specific region of DNA that is associated with these quantitative phenotypic traits. The number of QTLs that explain the variation in the phenotypic trait tells us more about the genetic structure of a specific trait. For example, the research related to QTLs could provide further information about the genes that control human height.

2.1.2 xQTL: Various types of QTL mapping

Microarray technology has elucidated the genetics of gene expression in human populations. It has been less successful to identify genes in underlying diseases by using molecular profiling tools. Since too many genes have been identified to be associated with disease traits, determining and verifying which genes are the true disease-causing genes have been difficult.

Recently, microarray techniques have been combined with genotyping technology to facilitate the identification of key drivers of complex diseases. Figure 1 represents this approach, treating relative transcript abundances as quantitative traits when segregating populations. In this method, chromosomal regions that control the level of expression of a particular gene are mapped as expression quantitative trait loci (eQTL).

This eQTL scheme can be easily extended to other data types, for example, proteome, metabolome and phenome. Figure 2 illustrates this extension: protein expression (pQTL), relative metabolites abundances (mQTL) and phenotype abundances (phQTL).

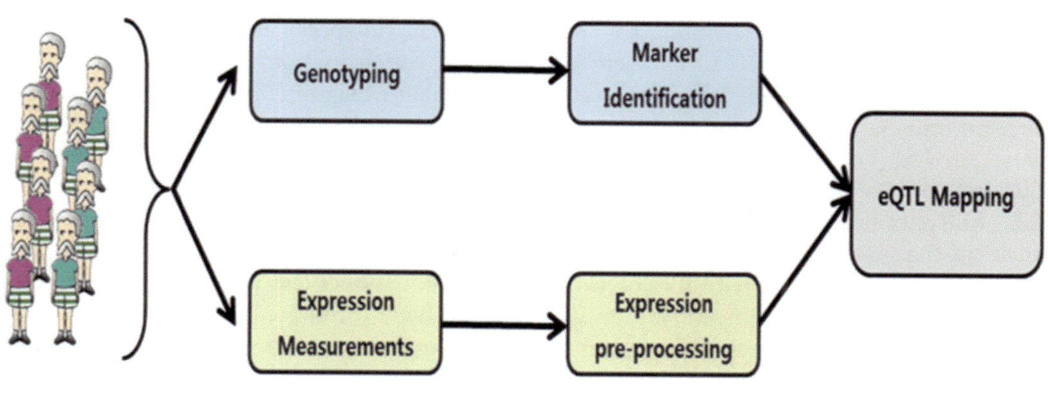

Fig. 1. eQTL pipeline. From disease and normal individuals, genotypes and mRNA expressions are observed.

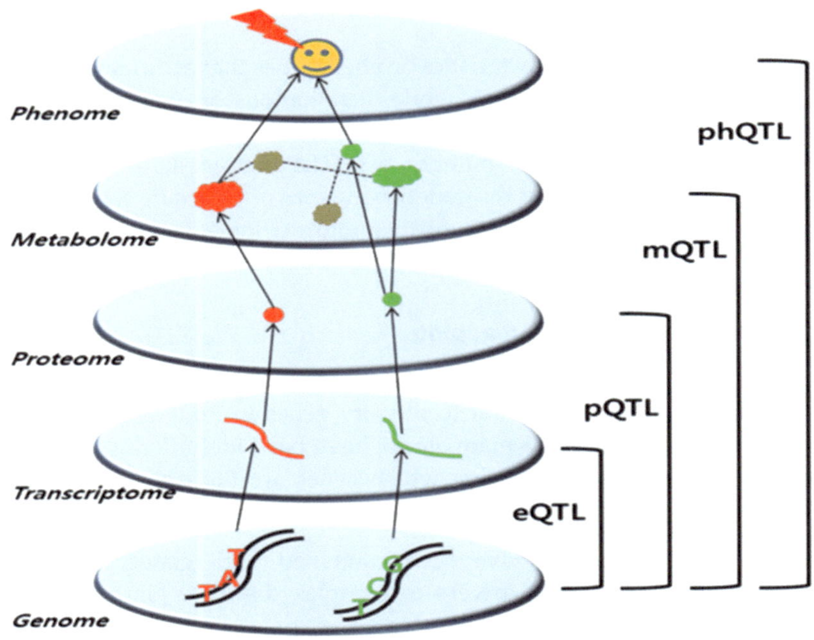

Fig. 2. A schematic representation of extended xQTL analyses.

2.2 Integrative analysis

Fu *et al.* provided the first system-wide evidence for phenotypic buffering in *Arabidopsis* [Fu *et al.*, 2009]. Their approach consisted of three steps. Step 1 performed QTL mapping for transcript, protein, metabolite and phenotypic trait data. Then, Step 2 computed significance thresholds for detection of QTL hotspots per level, and finally, Step 3 detected hotspots that appeared across multiple levels. In particular, at Step 2 permutation analysis was used to compute significance thresholds for detecting QTL hotspots. For each of the 250 permutations, all > 40,000 traits were analyzed in order to map QTLs and the most significant marker for each QTL was stored. The number of significnat QTLs were counted over all traits for each marker, and the significant thresholds for hotspot detection per level were derived. For system-wide or multiple level QTL hotspots, Step 3 used the observed QTL hotspots and permutation analysis to compute significance thresholds for detecting QTL hotspots that appeared at multiple levels. Using the results obtained from per-level analysis, the markers per level were ranked from the one with the highest number of traits mapping to it, to the one with the lowest. Then, a rank-product test was performed to find markers that ranked significantly high at multiple levels [Breitling *et al.*, 2004]. For each permutated sample, the *p*-value was computed for the rank-product test at each of the 144 markers, and a threshold was derived for hotspot detection by the procedure controlling 5% of the false discovery rate (FDR) [Benjamini & Hochberg, 1995].

Using this approach, 162 recombinant inbred lines (RIL) of *Arabidopsis thaliana* were profiled for variation in transcript, protein and metabolite abundance, and were mapped to QTL for 40,580 of these molecular traits. Only six QTL hotspots were found which underlied variation in 16% of the transcript traits, 25% of the protein traits, 55% of the metabolite traits and 77% of the phenotypic traits for which QTL could be mapped. QTL for 16%, 25%, 55% of all transcript, protein and metabolite traits with a QTL, respectively, mapped to the same six QTL hot spots, compared to 77% of phenotypic traits. Consequently, screening for mutants at the molecular level would increase the probability of identifying new causal loci that could not be identified from morphological screens [Boerjan & Vuylsteke, 2009].

Using microarrays or massively parallel sequencing it is possible to measure both genetic variation and gene expression at genomic level. Hence, eQTL methods allow for studying the association of all regions in a genome with the expression of all genes. In this sense it is worth re-visiting eQTL in deeper look.

If the genotype at a certain locus is associated with the phenotype of a certain gene, this DNA region might contain a regulator of the target gene expression. It could be any functional nucleotide sequences such as protein-coding regions, microRNAs and *cis*-regulatory DNA motifs. The same individuals of a selected population have to be genotyped and phenotyped first. Based on the genotyped data (*e.g.* SNP), selecting markers that are polymorphic in the study population is in need. Then, at the heart of every eQTL study is the correlation of genotype patterns with expression levels in a genetically diverse population. The simplest mapping strategy is to split the population based on the genotypes at a specific marker and check if the expression levels of a given gene are significantly different between the two groups [Ghazalpour *et al.*, 2008; Brem *et al.*, 2002; Kang *et al.*, 2008].

There have been many approaches to elucidate the variants affecting phenotypes, for example, Lan *et al.* explored correlation of expression profiles across a genetic dimension, namely genotypes segregating in a panel of 60 F_2 mice derived from a cross used to explore diabetes in obese mice. By combining the correlation results with linkage mapping information, they identified regulatory networks, made functinoal predictions for uncharacterized genes, and charaterized novel elements of knwon pathways [Lan *et al.*, 2006]. However, their approach did not provide any information about causality relationships among expression profile, genotype and disease.

The mixture over markers (MOM) model proposed by Kendziorski *et al.* combinds a transcript-based (TB) approach, refering to the repeated application of any single-phenotype mapping method to each mRNA transciprt, and a marker-based (MB) approach, refering to the repeated application, at each marker, of any method for identifying differnetially expressed transciprts [Kendziorski *et al.*, 2006]. They applied two MB approches: an empirical Bayes approach and an approach based on the Student's *t*-test. The MOM model is motivated from the fact that separate tests are conducted for each trascript-marker pair, and each measures evidence that the transcipt maps to that marker relative to evidence that it maps nowhere. Since a trancript can map to any of various marker locations, the evidence that a transcript maps to a particular marker should not be judged relative only to the possibility that it maps nowhere, but rather relative to the possibility that it maps nowhere or to some other markers. This model was proved useful in improving the specificity of eQTL identifications, but used only genotype variation and gene expressino data rather than disease status or trait data.

A gene-set approach based on weighted gene co-expression network analysis (WGCNA) by Presson *et al.* constructs a co-expression network, identifies trait-related modules within the network, uses a trait-related genetic marker to prioritize genes within the module, applies an integrated gene screening strategy to identify candidate genes and carries out causality testing to verify and/or prioritize results [Presson *et al.*, 2008]. Their work includes steps to identify trait-module association and trait-related genetic marker association, but does not provide the model-based statistical tests.

The step-wise approach proposed by Schadt *et al.* includes i) identifying pair-wise relationships among genotype variation, gene expression, and a complex trait, respectively investigated by identifying QTLs for the complex trait, ii) selecting gene expression traits correlated with the complex trait, iii) detecting eQTL, which overlap the identified QTL, for the selected expression traits; and iv) the likelihood based causality model selection (LCMS) test to identify the causal relationships of the genes detected with overlapping loci [Schadt *et al.*, 2005].

3. Two-step integrative analysis

Schadt *et al.*'s approah has two major limitations. First, although the filtering step is effective in reducing the search-space, it might result in more false negatives than exhaustive search approahes in detecting causal relationships of the genes, espeically when a true causal relationship exists based on the interaction effects among genotype, gene expression and a trait of interest, but any pairwise association is weak. Second, the model does not comprehensively handle the interaction effects, which might cause different disease susceptibility. Therefore Lee *et al.* proposed a two-step integrative approach handling with exhaustive search and interaction effects based on LCMS test [Lee *et al.*, 2009]. In this section we provide a detailed review of the Lee *et al.*'s two-step procedure integrating genotype data, gene expression and clinical data, and thus elucidating mechanisms underlying disease susceptibility and progression [Lee *et al*, 2009].

3.1 Introduction

In figure 3, the two-step procedure is presented to illustrate the integration method based on causal relationship among the three different levels of data. In the first step, the most appropriate causality models are selected to understand the causal relationship among genetic variation, gene expression level, and disease for each gene expression-genetic variation combination. In the second step, significance testing is carried out based on a

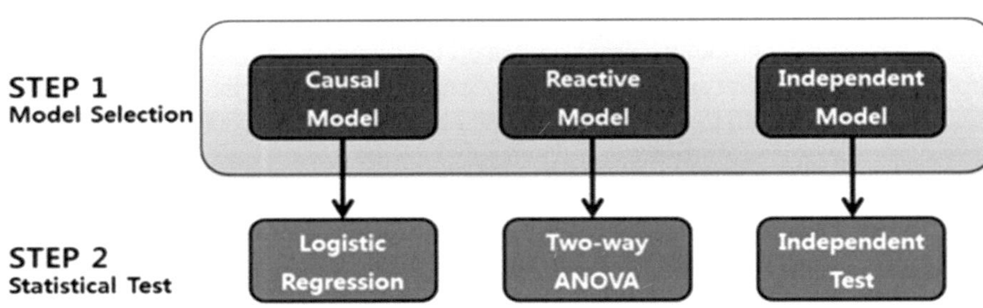

Fig. 3. Two-step procedure illustration of Lee *et al.'s*. In the first step, for each gene expression-genetic variation combination, the most appropriate causality models are selected. Then in the second step, significance test is carried out based on a statistical model for each combination according to the model selected in previous step.

statistical model for each combination, such as logistic regression and a two-way analysis of variance (ANOVA), according to the causality model selected from the first step. Through these tests, gene expression traits whose effects on disease status or responses to disease status are modified by the genotype variation effects.

3.2 The first step: Causality model selection

The possible causal relationships among genetic variation, gene expression level and disease trait, can be summarized as three models. Figure 4 represents three simple models. Causal model assumes the simplest causal relationship with respect to mRNA expression, in which QTL acts on disease through transcript. Reactive model is the model with respect to mRNA expression, in which mRNA expression is modulated by disease. In independent model, QTL at a specific locus acts on these traits independently.

Lee *et al.* assumed that each pair of genetic locus and expressed gene has one of these three simple causal relationships to examine potential relationships among the genotype variation, gene expression level and disease status. In order to find the most possible causal relation, both Lee *et al.* and Schadt *et al.* adapted the likelihood based causality model

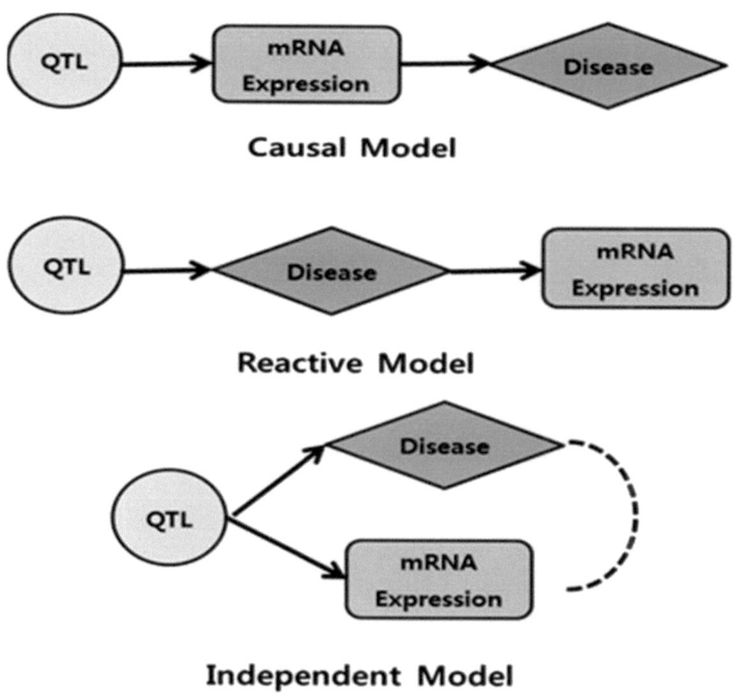

Fig. 4. Three possible causal relationships among genotype variation, mRNA level and complex disease proposed by Schadt *et al.* QTL, mRNA and disease represent any genotype variation like SNP, mRNA expression level of a gene, and complex disease or phenotype of interest, respectively.

selection (LCMS) test, which uses conditional correlation measures for determining the relationships best supported by the data. Unlike multistep procedure of Schadt *et al.*'s method, Lee *et al.* constructed likelihoods associated with each of the causality model and maximized with respect to the model parameters. Then, the best model was selected for each SNP-transcript combination, by choosing the model with the smallest Akaike Information Criterion (AIC) value which can be used to compare different models [Akaike, 1974).

Lee *et al.* and Schadt *et al.* both assumed standard Markov properties for the simple graphs (Fig. 4), the joint probability distributions for the three models are as follows:

- Causal Model: $P(S, R, D) = P(S)P(R|S)P(D|R)$,
- Reactive Model: $P(S, R, D) = P(S)P(D|S)P(R|D)$,
- Independent Model: $P(S, R, D) = P(S)P(R|S)P(D|R, S)$,

where S represents a genotype variation, R gene expression, and D disease status. P(S) is the genotype probability distribution for marker S and is further assumed to be co-dominant. $P(R\,|\,S)$ and $P(R\,|\,D)$ are the conditional probabilities of R given genotypes S and disease status D, respectively. Lee *et al.* further assumed that the random variable R follows conditional normal distribution, and the random variable D has a binomial distribution. Therefore, in probability $P(D\,|\,R)$, the random variable D has a binominal distribution with a success probability that can be modeled by a logistic regression model. $P(D\,|\,S)$ is the probability distribution of D conditional on locus S, in which the random variable D also has a binomial distribution. Based on these assumptions, the likelihood of a correspondence to each of the joint probability distributions can be constructed. For each model, the model parameters can be estimated via a standard maximum likelihood method. The best model supported by the data is then chosen based on the AIC, which is commonly used to compare models with different numbers of parameters [Schadt *et al.*, 2005; Lee *et al.* 2009]

3.3 The second step: Statistical test

Step 2 performs statistical tests to determine the significance of the genetic regulatory relationships described in the causality model selected at step 1. The response and independent variables in the statistical models depend on the causality model selected at step 1. These statistical tests can deal with the interaction effects among the three different levels of data and to elucidate differences in disease susceptibility and gene expression pattern across genetically different individuals. The two-step procedure can result in a set of candidate causal and reactive genes, whose expressions affect disease status and respond to disease status under the influence of genotype variation, respectively.

3.3.1 The causal model

In order to investigate gene expression traits whose effects on disease status are modified by genotype variation, the interaction effect of genotype variation and gene expression level on the disease status can be examined using logistic regression below:

$$\log\text{it}(\pi) = S + R + S \times R, \tag{1}$$

where π represents the probability of getting the disease; S represents the effect of genotype variation such as SNPs; R represents the effect of gene expression levels; and S × R represents the interaction effect between genotype variation and gene expression level.

3.3.2 The reactive model

For investigating gene expression traits whose responses to disease status are affected by genotype variations, one can fit the following two-way ANOVA model with the interaction between genotype variation and disease groups:

$$R = S + D + S \times D, \qquad (2)$$

where S represents the effect of genotype variation; D represents the effect of disease groups; and S × D represents the interaction effect between genotype variation and disease groups.

3.3.3 The independent model

When the independent model is selected at step 1, the effect of genotype variation on each of gene expression and disease can be investigated separately. First, the logistic regression is employed to detect genotypic markers linked to disease loci:

$$\log\text{it}(\pi) = S. \qquad (3)$$

Next, it is possible to identify genotypic markers that regulate gene expression levels, based on the one-way ANOVA model where the dependent variable is R and the independent variable is S.

In step 2, significant associations among genotype variation, gene expression and disease status are declared via statistical tests for all possible pairs of gene expression-genotype variation. Due to the large number of tests, the multiple-testing problem needs to be addressed. In order to adjust this multiplicity, Lee *et al.* used a step-up procedure controlling false discovery rate (FDR) [Benjamini & Hochberg, 1995].

4. Application

Lee *et al.* applied their two-step procedure to chronic fatigue syndrome (CFS) data to elucidate a list of potential causal genes of CFS. In this section, we provide the application of two-step procedure of Lee *et al.*'s

4.1 Chronic Fatigue Syndrome (CFS) dataset

Chronic fatigue syndrome (CFS) is a debilitating illness lacking consistent anatomic lesions and eluding conventional laboratory diagnosis. CFS has no confirmatory physical signs or laboratory abnormalities, and its etiology and pathophysiology are unknown. This disease characterized by chronic fatigue, lasting at least 6 months, which is accompanied by symptoms such as impairment in short-term memory or concentration, sore throat, tender lymph nodes, and muscle pain. The Centers for Disease Control and Prevention (CDC) Chronic Fatigue Syndrome Research Group produced the dataset including gene expression of 177 subjects, proteomic of 60 subjects, single nucleotide polymorphism (SNP) of 50 subjects, and clinical data of 227 subjects. All the data set is available on the following web site (*http://www.camda.duke.edu/camda06/datasets/index.html*).

According to severity of symptoms, the patients were originally classified into five groups of CFS. Lee *et al.*'s study, however, only consider three groups of total 101 subjects: 46 subjects meeting the CFS research case definition (CFS), 19 subjects meeting the CFS research case definition and having 'a major depressive disorder with melancholic features' (CFS-MDD/m), and 36 subjects who show no fatigue (NF).

This CFS dataset has been analysed by many research groups for identifying molecular markers and elucidating pathophysiology of CFS, for finding two differentially expressed genes related with fatigue and depression, respectively, for discriminating classes of unexplained chronic fatigue based on differential gene expressions, and for examining the relationship between CFS and allostatic load based on the clinical dataset. In the CFS dataset, the expression levels of 20,160 genes were assessed from peripheral blood mononuclear cells, via custom-printed single-channel oligonucleotide chips. Quantile normalization was conducted on the gene expression data which were pre-processed by the original CDC research group. For genotype data, the whole blood DNA was extracted and specific areas of the genes of interest were amplified by PCR.

For illustration, we summarized the analyses results from the multi-step procedure of Schadt *et al.* and the two-step approach of Lee *et al.* The detailed description of the results is provided in Lee *et al.* [Lee *et al.*, 2009].

4.2 Results

4.2.1 Multi-step procedure by Schadt *et al.*

The multi-step procedure proposed by Schadt *et al.* was applied to the same datasets for the purpose of comparison. First, a gene expression analysis was carried out to detect differentially expressed genes across clinical outcomes. Only a few genes were identified as differentially expressed (Table 1A) by three commonly used approaches such as the t-test, significance analysis of microarray (SAM) [Tusher *et al.*, 2001] and the Bayesian regression approach [Baldi & Long, 2001]. Second, genotype variation data and clinical outcomes were analyzed via logistic regression to detect the susceptibility genes of disease. Out of all 41 markers tested, nine markers were detected with significant genotype effect on initiation of CFS at a 5% significance level, while only four markers were detected with 5% FDR [Benjamini & Hochberg, 1995] (Table 1B). Interestingly, different sets of susceptible genes were identified as having statistically significant association with CFS and CFS-MDD/m. From the CFS vs. NF comparison, the seven markers in the NR3C1 gene were identified as significant markers linked to CFS. On the other hand, the CFS-MDD/m vs. NF comparison revealed the two significant markers in the COMT gene. Finally, for each of the differentially expressed genes across clinical outcomes, eQTL were searched at each of the markers that were identified at the second step, via one-way ANOVA of genotype variation and gene expression data. No significant association between gene expression level and genotype variation was found for any genotype–gene expression combination at a 5% significant level.

Dataset	*t*-test	SAM test	Bayesian model
A. Number of genes with significant change in expression levels over different disease status, which were detected via *t*-test, SAM test and Bayesian model.			
CFS vs. NG	1	2	0
CFS-MDD/m vs. NF	1	1	0

Gene	SNP[a]	Chromosome	Position(Mb)[b]	CFS vs. NF	CFS-MDD/m vs. NF[c]
B Significant genotype variation linked to disease loci, which were detected via logistic regression					
NR3C1[e]	rs2918419	5	142.641	0.0104	0.3950
	rs1866388	5	142.702	0.0010[f]	0.0472
	rs860458	5	142.739	0.0104	0.3950
	rs852977	5	146.642	0.0035[f]	0.1878
	rs6196	5	146.660	0.0208	0.6423
	rs6188	5	146.667	0.0027[f]	0.0396
	rs258750	5	146.674	0.0035[f]	0.1009
COMT[g]	rs933271	22	18.311	0.0649	0.0025
	rs5993882	22	18.317	0.4306	0.0114

Table 1. parallel analyses for respective association of gene expression and genotype variation with disease status (by courtesy of the authors) [Lee *et al.*, 2009]

As multiple filtering steps is Schadt et al.'s procedure, the separate analyses were conducted respectively on two datasets, CFS vs. NF groups and CFS-MDD/m vs. NF groups. Bold numbers indicate *p*-values < 0.05.

[a] NCBI dbSNP Build number is 125 using Human Genome Build 35.1

[b] Position of SNP on chromosome.1

[c] *p*-value from logistic regression with CFS vs. NF data.

[d] *p*-value from logistic regression with CFS-MDD/m vs. NF data.

[e] Glucocorticoid receptor located at 5q34.

[f] Significant at the 5% false discovery rate (FDR).

[g] Catechol-O-methyltransferase located at 22q11.1.

In other words, no significant results were detected for both datasets from the Schadt *et al.*'s multi-step method.

4.2.2 Two-step integrative analysis

Lee *et al.* analyzed each combination of 20,160 genes and 41 SNPs with their two-step integrative analysis on two datasets, CFS vs. NF groups and CFS-MDD/m vs. NF groups. For each gene–SNP combination, the best causal relationship was detected via the causality model selection at step 1. In comparing CFS with NF groups, the reactive model was selected for ~70% of 20,160 genes on average, for all nine markers within two known CFS-related genes, such as NR3C1 and COMT (Table 2). However, in comparing CFS-MDD/m with NF groups, the causal model was selected for nearly 70% genes for three markers in the NR3C1 gene. This different tendency in the model selection results between CFS and CFS-MDD/m would imply different genetic mechanisms of CFS and CFS-MDD/m.

At step 2, each gene–SNP combination data was analyzed based on one of the three statistical models, corresponding to the detected causal relationship. For all seven SNPs within NR3C1, significant causal relationships with gene expression levels were detected for either or both datasets (Table 2). Three SNPs (rs258750, rs6188 and rs852977) showed significant relationships with expression levels of a large number of genes, and can be candidates for genetic modulators of CFS- related regulatory pathways.

Gene	SNP	CFS vs. NF			CFS-MDD/m vs. NF		
		Causal[a]	Reactive[b]	Independent[c]	Causal[a]	Reactive[b]	Independent[c]
NR3C1[d]	Rs2918419	0 (639)	7 (16,215)	0 (3306)	8 (13,955)	3 (5912)	0 (293)
	Rs1866388	0 (165)	0 (16,872)	0 (3123)	15 (4136)	71 (15,976)	0 (48)
	Rs860458	0 (639)	7 (16,215)	0 (3306)	8 (13,955)	3 (5912)	0 (293)
	Rs852977	0 (230)	0 (17,001)	0 (2929)	**120 (9760)**	**73 (10,139)**	**0 (261)**
	Rs6196	0 (604)	2 (15,037)	0 (4519)	0 (16,278)	0 (2013)	0 (1869)
	Rs6188	0 (171)	7 (16,970)	1 (3019)	**52 (2939)**	**217 (17,074)**	**0 (147)**
	Rs258750	**0 (242)**	**0 (16,279)**	**105 (3639)**	0 (2769)	14 (12,590)	0 (4801)
COMT[e]	Rs933271	0 (1943)	0 (15,156)	0 (3061)	0 (169)	0 (16,872)	0 (3119)
	Rs5993882	0 (1022)	0 (14,380)	0 (4758)	0 (547)	0 (17,333)	0 (2280)

Table 2. Two-step integration based on causality model selection. (by courtesy of the authors) [Lee *et al.*, 2009]

The integrative analyses were conducted respectively on two datasets, CFS vs. NF groups and CFS-MDD/m vs. NF groups. Note that the results are presented only for nine SNPs within two known CFS-related genes (NR3C1 and COMT). For each combination of 20,160 genes and 41 SNPs, the best causal relationship was detected via causal model selection at step 1. Numbers in parenthesis indicate the numbers of genes having each causal relationship with each SNP and disease status. At step 2, each gene-SNP combination data was analyzed based on one of the three statistical models, corresponding to the detected causal relationship. Outside parenthesis, we present the numbers of significant genes identified by the corresponding statistical models. Three SNPs, each of which involves significant causal relationships with expression levels of more than 100 genes, are marked in bold.

[a] Logistic regression was conducted to identify genes whose expressions have interaction effect with genotype variation on disease status.

[b] Two-way ANOVA was conducted to identify genes whose expressions are affected by interaction between genotype variation and disease status.

[c] Independent test was conducted to identify genes whose expressions differ according to SNP genotypes.

[d] Gluccorticoid receptor located at 5q34.

[e] Catechol-O-methltransferase located at 22q11.1.

Next, pathway enrichment analyses were performed for these three SNPs, and the results are given in the next section. In comparing CFS with NF groups, for the rs258750 marker, 105 genes were identified with differential expression across genotypes with 5% FDR from the independent test. This result is supported by the evidence of the neuroendocrine regulation of immunity, because the gene expression data were obtained from a mononuclear cell, and the role of glucocorticoid receptor (NR3C1) gene is to regulate the level of glucocorticoid.

In the integrated analysis for comparing CFS-MDD/m with NF groups, for the rs6188 marker in the NR3C1 gene, 52 genes showed significant interaction effects with the rs6188 marker on disease status CFS-MDD/m from the logistic regression model. Also, the two-way ANOVA models yielded 217 candidate reactive genes, on which there are significant interaction effects between disease status and genotypes. Note that these candidate genes, especially reactive genes, could not be detected by Schadt *et al.*'s method. The Lee *et al.*'s two-step integration method revealed the causal association among gene expression level, genotype and disease status in depth. Candidate causal/reactive genes were detected also for rs852977 in the NR3C1 gene. However, the candidate gene set for the rs852977 is very similar to that for the rs6188, with slight differences in causality structure. This similarity would be due to a strong linkage between the two SNPs.

4.2.3 Pathway enrichment analysis

In comparing CFS with NF groups, Lee *et al.* further conducted a pathway enrichment analysis for 105 genes that were identified to have a significant relationship with the rs258750 marker from the independent test at step 2. The pathway classification showed that nine different pathways were associated with the rs258750 marker at the 5% significance level (Table 3). Out of nine pathways, four were enriched with genes involved in regulation of transcription, translation or mRNA processing, and three are related with immune system.

For comparing CFS-MDD/m with NF groups, pathway enrichment analyses were conducted on the genes that were identified to have a significant relationship with the rs6188 and/or rs852977 markers at step 2. Because of the linkage between the two SNPs, the results were similar (Tables 4 and 5), and the results was given only for the rs6188. While seven different pathways were detected at the 5% significance level for the 52 candidate causal genes, eleven different pathways were detected for the 217 candidate reactive genes (Table 4). In addition, two other pathways, whose p-values were slightly larger than the 5% significance level, are listed.

In pathway enrichment analyses of the candidate causal genes, the steroid biosynthesis pathway appears to have a direct causal effect on the disease status, CFS-MDD/m, through an integrative action of the rs6188 marker within the NR3C1 gene. The two significantly enriched biological pathways (i.e., 'IL-2 Receptor Beta Chain in T cell Activation', and 'HIV-1 Nef: negative effector of FAS and TNF') are all related to the immune system. On the other hand, the pathway enrichment analysis of the candidate reactive genes showed that several pathways related to lipid metabolism or biosynthesis, such as eicosanoid and fatty acid, appear to be important for responding to CFS-MDD/m. Furthermore, other pathways associated with neuron physiology and neurotransmitters appear to respond to CFS-MDD/m.

Pathway[a]	Model[b]	Source[c]	Nodes[d]	Gene ID [e]	Gene name
Galactose metabolism	Indepe-ndent	KEGG	2/22	B4GALT2 MGAM	UDP-Gal:betaGlcNAc beta 1,4-galactosyltransferase, polypeptide2 Maltase-glucoamylase
Basic mechanisms of SUMOylation	Indepe-ndent	BioCarta	1/4	SUMO3	SMT3 suppressor of mif two 3 homolog 3
Internal ribosome entry pathway	Indepe-ndent	BioCarta	1/8	EIF4E	Eukaryotic translation initiation factor 4E
Neutrophil and its surface molecules	Indepe-ndent	BioCarta	1/8	ITGB2	Integrin, beta 2
Alternative complement pathwy	Indepe-ndent	BioCarta	1/9	CFB	Complement factor B
Mechanisms of protein import into the nucleus	Indepe-ndent	BioCarta	1/9	NUP62	Nucleoporin 62kDa
Polyadenylation of mRNA	Indepe-ndent	BioCarta	1/9	PABP2	Poly(A) binding protein II
B Lymphocyte cell surface molecules	Indepe-ndent	BioCarta	1/9	ITGB2	Integrin, beta 2
Adhesion molecules on lymphocyte	Indepe-ndent	BioCarta	1/9	ITGB2	Integrin, beta 2

Table 3. Significant regulated pathways for SNP rs258750 (by courtesy of the authors) [Lee *et al.*, 2009]

Pathway enrichment analysis was conducted using 105 candidate independent genes, which were identified for rs258750. Significant biological pathways were detected via Fisher's exact test at a 5% significance level. Pathways are listed in order of significance e.g., most significant pathway presents at the top.

[a] Name of biological pathway selected by Fisher's exact test.

[b] Causality models selected ay step1.

[c] Source of pathway

[d] The number of candidate causal/reactive genes associated with pathway/the number of all genes associated with pathway.

[e] Gene ID of candidate genes associated with pathway

Pathway[a]	Model[b]	Source[c]	Nodes[d]	Gene ID [e]	Gene name
Electron transport chain	Causal	GenMapp	2/105	COX11 COX6A1	Cytochrome c oxidase subunit11 Cytochrome c oxidase subunit Via polypeptide 1
Steroid biosynthesis	Causal	GenMapp	1/9	F13B	Coagulation factor XIII,B polypeptide
Blood clotting cascade	Causal	GenMapp	1/19	F13B	Coagulation factor XIII,B polypeptide
FAS signaling pathway(CD95)	Causal	BioCarta	1/30	CFLAR	CASP8 and FADD-like apoptosis regulator
Induction of apoptosis through DR3 and DR4/5 Death Receptor	Causal	BioCarta	1/32	CFLAR	CASP8 and FADD-like apoptosis regulator
IL-2 receptor beta chain in T cell activation	Causal	BioCarta	1/35	CFLAR	CASP8 and FADD-like apoptosis regulator
HIV-1 Nef:negative effector of FAS and TNF	Causal	BioCarta	1/57	CFLAR	CASP8 and FADD-like apoptosis regulator
Agrin in postsynaptic differentiation	Reactive	BioCarta	3/39	UTRN DVL1 ARHGEF6	Utrophin Dishevelled,dsh homolog1 Rac/Cdc42 guanine nucleotide exchange factor(GEF)6
Cell cycle	Reactive	GenMapp	4/87	CDC14A E2F2 CDC20	CDC14 cell division cycle 20homolog E2F transcription factor2 CDC20 cell division cycle 20homolog
Eicosanoid metabolism	Reactive	BioCarta	2/20	PTGES EPHX1	Prostaglandin E synthase Epoxide hydrolase
Biosyntheisis of cysteine	Reactive	BioCarta	1/2	CBS	Cystathionine-beta-synthase
Biosyntheisis of threonine and methionine	Reactive	BioCarta	1/2	CBS	Cystathionine-beta-synthase

Pathway[a]	Model[b]	Source[c]	Nodes[d]	Gene ID [e]	Gene name
Inactivation of Gsk3 by AKT causes accumulation of β-catenin in alveolar macrophages	Reactive	BioCarta	2/25	MYD88 DVL1	Myeloid differentiation primary response gene (88) Disheveled, dsh homolog 1
Fatty acid metabolism	Reactive	KEGG	3/57	HADHB	Hydroxyacyl-Coenzyme A dehydrogenase/3-ketoacyl-Coenzyme A thiolase/enoyl-Coenzyme A hydraatase, beta subunit
Bile acid biosynthesis	Reactive	KEGG	2/26	ADH6	Alcohol dehydrogenase 6 (class V)
Catabolic pathways for methionine,isoleucine,threonine And valine	Reactive	BioCarta	1/4	CBS	Cystathionie-beta-synthase
Basic mechanisms of SUMOylation	Reactive	BioCarta	1/4	SMT3H1	SMT3 suppressor of mif two 3 homolog 3
ALK in cardiac myocytes	Reactive	BioCarta	2/34	DLV1 CHRD	Chordin
Taurine and hypotaurine metabolism[f]	Reactive	KEGG	1/5	GAD1	Glutamate decarboxylase 1
Biosynthesis of neurotransmitters[f]	Reactive	BioCarta	1/6	GAD1	Glutamate decarboxylase 1

Table 4. Significant regulated pathways for SNP rs6188 (by courtesy of the authors) [Lee *et al.*, 2009]

Pathway enrichment analysis was conducted using 52 candidate causal genes and 217 candidate reactive genes, which were identified for rs6188. Significant biological pathways were detected via Fisher's exact test at a 5% significance level. Pathways are listed in order of significance within each of causality models, e.g., most significant pathway presents at the top.

[a] Name of biological pathway selected by Fisher's exact test.

[b] Causality models selected ay step1.

[c] Source of pathway

[d] The number of candidate causal/reactive genes associated with pathway/the number of all genes associated with pathway.

[e] Gene ID of candidate genes associated with pathway.

[f] Pathways with *p*-value that is slightly larger than 0.05.

Pathway[a]	Model[b]	Source[c]	Nodes[d]	Gene ID [e]	Gene name
Agrin in postsynaptic differentiation	Causal	BioCarta	2/39	DMD DVL1	Dystrophin Dishevelled, dsh homolog 1
Steroid biosynthesis	Causal	Gen MAPP	1/9	F13B	Coagulation factor XIII, B polypeptide
Nucleotide GPCRs	Causal	Gen MAPP	1/10	P2RY4	Pyrimidinergic receptor P2Y, G-protein coupled 4
RNA polymerase III transcription	Causal	BioCarta	1/8	GTF3C1	General transcription factor IIIC, polypeptide 1, alpha 220kDa
Blood clotting cascade	Causal	Gen MAPP	1/19	F13B	Coagulation factor XIII, B polypeptide
Bile acid biosynthesis	Causal	KEGG	1/26	ADH6	Alcohol dehydrogenase 6
Tyrosine metabolism	Causal	KEGG	1/37	ADH6	Alcohol dehydrogenase 6I
Inactivation of Gsk3 by AKT causes accumulation of b-catenin in alverolar macrophages	Reactive	BioCarta	1/25	MYD88 DVL1	Myeloid differentiation primary response gene (88) Dishevelled, dsh homolog 1
ALK in cardiac myocytes	Reactive	BioCarta	1/34	DVL1 CHRD	Dishevelled, dsh homolog 1 Chordin
Biosynthesis of neurotransmitter	Reactive	BioCarta	1/6	GAD1	Glutamate decarboxylase 1
Taurine and hypotaurine metabolism	Reactive	KEGG	1/5	GAD1	Glutamate decarboxylase 1
Electron transport chain	Reactive	Gen MAPP	2/105	COX11 COX6A1	Cytochrome c oxidase subunit 11 Cytochrome c oxidase subunit Vla polypeptide 1

Table 5. Significant regulated pathways for SNP rs852977 (by courtesy of the authors) [Lee *et al.*, 2009]

Pathway enrichment analysis was conducted using 120 candidate causal genes, which were identified for rs852977. Significant biological pathways were detected via Fisher's exact test at a 5% significance level. Pathways are listed in order of significance within each of causality model, e.g., most significant pathway presents at the top.

[a] Name of biological pathway selected by Fisher's exact test.

[b] Causality models selected ay step1.

[c] Source of pathway

[d] The number of candidate causal/reactive genes associated with pathway/the number of all genes associated with pathway.

[e] Gene ID of candidate genes associated with pathway.

5. Discussion

The two-step procedure can integrate gene expression data, genotype variation data and clinical data, and identify the genetic mechanism of a complex disease. We described three different statistical tests based on the two-step procedure proposed by Lee *et al.*. For purposes of comparison, two different CFS related datasets were analyzed via the multi-step procedure proposed by Schadt *et al.*. In these specific datasets, no significant results were detected from the multistep method of Schadt *et al.*, while the method of Lee *et al.* enabled us to identify many statistically significant causal relationships, some of which were biologically supported by pathway enrichment analyses. These results demonstrated that the two-step method based on an exhaustive search investigation would provide more power.

Furthermore, the two-step approach provided some interesting results. First, CFS groups and CFS-MDD/m groups would appear to have different genotypes and gene expression profiles even though they had the common characteristic of chronic fatigue. In particular, CFS has major susceptibility markers within the NR3C1 gene, and CFSMDD/m seems to have major susceptibility markers within the catechol-O-methyltransferase (COMT) gene, though they are not statistically significant after FDR correction (Table 1B). The NR3C1 gene regulates the level of glucocorticoid which is the end product of the hypothalamic-pituitary-adrenal (HPA) whereas COMT catalyzes the transfer of a methyl group from S-adenosylmethionine to catecholamines, which is the principal end product of the sympathetic nervous system (SNS), of which the role is maintaining stress-related homeostasis [Elenkov *et al.,* 2000]. The different major susceptibility gene may be related with to the provoking of MDD/m.

Second, polymorphisms in the glucocorticoid receptor NR3C1 gene act on CFS and CFS-MDD/m differently. The polymorphisms (rs258750) within NR3C1 have significant effects on CFS, and the 105 gene expression levels independently. However, in the integrated analysis for comparing CFS-MDD/m and NF groups, polymorphisms within the NR3C1 gene affect the CFS-MDD/m and several gene expression levels differently. For example, the 217 genes are differentially expressed according to the rs6188 marker genotype within NR3C1 and disease status, even though polymorphisms within NR3C1 have no direct significant effects after FDR correction on the CFS-MDD/m. In addition, the 52 genes also regulate the CFS-MDD/m, through integrated action with the rs6188 marker. The different action of the NR3C1 gene on gene expression level and disease may be an outcome of other factors, such as environmental effects or polymorphisms of the COMT gene. The catecholamines which are regulated by the COMT gene, have been often been regarded as immunosuppressive [Elenkov *et al.,* 2000].

Two pathway enrichment analyses for the 52 candidate causal genes and 217 candidate reactive genes indicated that our approach can recover plausible regulatory mechanisms of CFS-MDD/m by comparing CFS-MDD/m and NF groups. From the comparison, we noticed that the pathways related to the immune system and steroid may have causal effect on disease state through an integrative action of the NR3C1 gene. Both the NR3C1 gene that regulates the level of glucocorticoid, and the steroid that includes corticosteroids are known to regulate the immune function [Webster *et al.,* 2002]. A number of studies have found many irregularities in the immune systems in CFS patients [Natelson *et al.,* 2002]. This suggested that an important cause of CFS-MDD/m would be the immune system dysfunction, regulated by the neuroendocrine system, which rs6188 in the NR3C1 gene seems influence. Another potential implication of this comparison is that the CFS-MDD/m status and genetic polymorphisms can jointly induce different activation and expression of several lipid related metabolisms, neuron physiology differentiation, and neurotransmitters. Our results are supported by the known relationship between eicosanoid or fatty acid and CFS [Grey & Martinovic, 1994; Puri, 2007; Puri *et al.*, 2004; Liu *et al.*, 2003].

However, since fatigue is a core symptom in major depressive disorder [Pae *et al.*, 2007], CFS-MDD/m patients might have fatigue due to the depression rather than unexplained causes, and hence the significant results may be related to a 'major depression disorder with melancholic features' rather than chronic fatigue. For example, the excessive hypothalamus-pituitary-adrenal (HPA) axis responses, of which the end products are glucocorticoids, are known to be hallmarks of depression [Pariante & Miller, 2001; Holsboer, 2000; Pariante, 2004]. Also, the major depression can be associated with the immune activation, dysfunction of neurotransmitters at synapse [Neumeister *et al.*, 2004; Sanacora *et al.*, 2004; Maes & Meltzer, 1995], and essential fatty acids [Van Strater & Bouvy, 2006].

The integrative analyses considering the interaction effect among different levels of data could elucidate different disease susceptibility and differentially expressed genes of genetically different individuals. Some results showed that integrating genotype and expression data may help the search for new directions for the treatment of common human diseases that are not being detected using only one type of data. The integrated analysis provided more information than the two separate analyses of gene expression data and genotype variation data for characterizing CFS that has several possible causes.

In conclusion, the two-step approach to the integration of heterogeneous data sets can be generally applied to other studies in which gene expression data, genotype variation data and clinical data are available, and it can be very useful as the importance of integrated data analysis has been increasing. The two-step approach can also be extended to datasets containing other type of data, such as protein data rather than clinical data. The two-step approach can be readily applicable to quantitative traits rather than binary clinical outcome traits, by employing linear regression analysis. Also, it can be easily applied to genome-wide association studies, and can handle environmental factors, such as age and sex, by treating these factors as covariates in the regression model. Furthermore, the two-step approach can be extended to the gene-set approach, the module based approach or co-expression network as Presson *et al.* [Presson *et al.*, 2008] and Chen *et al.* [Chen *et al.*, 2008] did.

However, there are some limitations to the two-step method. First, the causality models are too simple to represent true mechanisms, which would be more complicated due to possible interactions between causal-reactive genes [Schadt *et al.*, 2005]. Further considerations for more complicated models are necessary in order to identify the genetic mechanism of complex diseases. Second, the two-step approach may need large computing although it is applicable to genome-wide studies because it is not limited in the scale of data. Another limitation would be a misclassification problem in that the proposed method relies on the LCMS. The current two-step approach does not use FDR procedure to account for the model misclassification problem. In fact, FDR procedure was employed only in the second step, not in the first step for the model selection procedure that chooses the model with the minimum

AIC among the three causal models. While anticipating the problem, we still employed the LCMS process because it showed good power for detecting true models in the simulation evaluated by Schadt *et al.* The two-step approach can be extended to account for the errors caused by the model misclassification in the first step. For example, we can test for the difference in the AIC values of three causality models, because the chance for model misclassification would be high when the difference between the smallest AIC value from the selected model and those from the other models is not large. A permutation-based nonparametric test might be developed for this testing. We think it requires a further study to control simultaneously two types of errors: causality model selection, and significant maker-gene pair identification.

6. Acknowledgment

The work was supported by the National Research Foundation (KRF-2008-313-C00086)

7. References

Akaike, H. (1974) A new look at the statistical model identification. *IEEE Transactions on Automatic Control.* Vol.19, pp.716-723

Baldi, P. & Long, A.D. (2001) A Bayesian Framework for the Analysis of Microarray Expression Data : regularized *t*-test and statistical inferences of gene changes. *Bioinformatics.* Vol.17, pp.509-519

Benjamini, Y. & Hochberg, Y. (1995). Controlling the False Discovery Rate - a pratical and powerful approach to multiple testing. *Journal of the Royal Statistical Society.* Vol.B57. pp.289-300

Boerjan, W. & Vuylsteke, M. (2009). Integrative genetical genomics in Arabidopsis. *Nature Genetics.* Vol.41, No.2, pp.144-145

Breitling, R. ; Armengaud, P. ; Amtmann, A. & Herzyk, P. (2004). Rank products : a simple, yet powerful, new method to detect differentially regulated genes in replicated microarray experiments. *FEBS Letters.* Vol.573, pp.83-92

Brem, R.B. ; Yvert, G.l ; Clinton, R. & Kruglyak, L. (2002). Genetic Dissection of Transcriptional Regulation in Budding Yeast. *Science.* Vol.296, pp.297-392

Chen, Y. ; Zhu, J. ; Lum, P.Y. ; Yang, X . ; Pinto, S. ; MacNeil, D.J. ; Zhang, C. ; Lamb, J. ; Edwards, S. ; Sieberts, S.K. ; Leonardson, A. ; Castellini, L.W. ; Wang, S. ; Champy, M.F. ; Zhang, B. ; Emilsson, V. ; Doss, S. ; Ghazalpour, A. ; Horvath, S. ; Drake, T.A. ; Lusis, A.J. & Schadt E.E. (2008). Variations in DNA Elucidate Molecular Networks That Cause Disease. *Nature.* Vol.452. pp.429-435

Coffey, C.S. ; Hebert, P.R. ; Ritchie, M.D. ; Krumholz, H.M. ; Gaziano, J.M. ; Ridker, P.M. ; Brown, N.J. ; Vaughan D.E. & Moore, J.H. (2004). An Application of Conditional Logistic Regression and Multifactor Dimensionality Reduction for Detecting Gene-Gene Interactions on Risk of Myocardial Infaction : The Importance of Model Validation. *BMC Bioinformatics.* Vol.5:49

Elenkov, J. ; Wilder, R.L. ; Chrousos, G.P. & Vizi, E.S. The sympathetic Nerve - an integrative interface between tow supersystems : the brain and the immune system. (2000). *Pharmacological Review.* Vol.52. pp. 595-638

Fu, J.; Keurentijes, J.J.B. ; Bouwmeester, H. ; America, T. ; Verstappen, F.W.A . ; Ward, J.L. ; Beale, M.H. ; Vos, R.C.H. ; Dijkstra, M. ; Scheltema, R.A. ; Johannes, F. ; Koornneef,

M. ; Vreugdenhil, D. ; Breitling, R. & Jansen, R.C. (2009). System-wide Molecular Evidence for Phenotypic Buffering in Arabidopsis, *Natrue Genetics,* Vol.41, No.2, pp. 166-167

Ghazalpour, A. ; Doss, S. ; Kang, H. ; Farber, C. ; Wen P.Z. ; Brozell, A. ; Castellanos, R. ; Eskin, E. ; Smith, D.J. ; Drake, T.A. & Lusis, A.J. (2008). High-Resolution Mapping of Gene Expression Using Association in an Outbred Mouse Stock. *PloS Genetics.* Vol.4, e100149.

Gray, J.B. & Martinovic, A.M. (1994) Eicosanoids and Essential Fatty-acid Modulation in Chornic Disease and the Chronic Fatigue Syndrome. *Med.Hypotheses.* Vol.43 pp.31-42

Henshall, J.M. ; Goddard, M.E. (1999) Multiple-Trait Mapping of Quantitative Trait Loci After Selective Genotyping Using Logistic Regression. *Genetics.* Vol.151, pp.885-894

Holsboer, F. (2000). The Corticosteroid Receptor Hypothesis of Depression. *Neuropsychopharmacology.* Vol.23. pp.477-501

Howell, W.M, ; Jobs, M. ; Gyllensten, U. & Brookes A.J. (1999). A New Method for Scoring Single Nucleotide Polymorphisms. *Nature Biotechnology.* Vol.17. pp.87-88

Jansen, R.C. (2009). Genetical Genomics Tutorial. Available from http://www.ipk-gatersleben.de/Internet/Forschung/Doktorandenprogramm/StudentBoard/Guest Speakers/Jansen_2009.pdf

Kang, H.M. ; Zaitlen, N.A. ; Wade, C.M. ; Kirby, A. ; Heckerman, D. ; Daly, M.J. & Eksin, E. (2008) Efficient Control of Population Structure in Model Organism Association Mapping. *Genetics.* Vol.178, pp.1709-1723

Kendziorski, C.M. ; Chen, M. ; Yuan, M. & Attie, L.A.D. (2006) Statistical Methods for Expression Quantitative Trait Loci (eQTL) mapping. *Biometrics.* Vol.62. pp.19-27

Lan, H. ; Chen, M. ; Flowers, J.B. ; Yandell, B.S. ; Stapleton, D.S. ; Mata, C.M. ; Mui, E.T. ; Flowers, M.T. ; Chueler, K.L. ; Manly, K.F. ; Williams, R.W. ; Kendziorski, C. & Attie, A.D. (2006). Combined Expression Trait Correlations and Expression Quantitative Trait Locus Mapping. *PloS Genetics.* Vol.2, e6

Lee, E.; Cho, S.; Kim, K. & Park T. (2009). An Integrated Approach to Infer Associations Among Genes Expression, Genotype Variation, and Disease. *Genomics.* Vol.94, pp.269-277

Lin, E & Hsu S. (2009). A Bayesian Approach to Gene-Gene and Gene-Environment Interactions in Chronic Fatigue Syndrome. *Pharmacogenomics.* Vol.10. pp.35-42

Liu, Z. ; Wang, D. ; Xue, Q. ; Chen, K. ; Bai, X. & Chang, L. (2003) Determinination of Fatty Acid Levels in Erythrocyte Membranes of Patients with Chronic Fatigue Syndrome. *Nutr. Neurosci.* Vol.6. pp.389-392

Maes, M. & Meltzer, H.Y. (1995) *The Serotonin Hypothesis of Major Depression.* Raven Press, New York

Michaelson, J.J. ; Loguercio, S. & Beyer, A. (2009). Detection and Interpretation of Expression QuantitativeTrait Loci (eQTL). *Methods.* Vol.48. pp.265-276

Natelson, B.H. ; Haghighi, M.H. & Ponzio, N.M. Evidence for the Presence of Immune Dysfunction in Chornic Fatigue Syndrome. (2002). *Clin. Diagn. Lab. Immunol.* Vol.9. pp.747-752

Neumeister, A.; Young, T. & Stastny, J. (2004). Implications of Genetic Research on the Role of the Serotonin in Depression: emphasis on the setotonin type 1(A) receptor and the serotonin transporter. *Psychopharmacology.* Vol.174. pp.512-524

Pae, C.U.; Lim, H.K.; Han, C.; Patkar, A.A.; Steffens, D.C.; Masand, P.S. & Lee, C. (2007) Fatigue as a Core Symptom in Major Depressive Disorder: overview and the role of bupropion. *Exper Rev. Neurotherapeutics*. Vol.7. pp.1251-1263

Pariante, C.M. (2004). Glucocorticoid Receptor Function in Vitro in Patients with Major Depression. *Stress*. Vol.7. pp.209-219

Pariante, C.M. & Miller, A.H. (2001). Glucocorticoid Recpetors in Major Depression: relevance to pathophysiology and treatment. *Biol. Phychiatry*. Vol.49. pp.391-404

Presson, A.P. ; Sobel, E.M. ; Papp, J.C. ; Suarez, C.J. ; Whistler, T. ; Rajeevan, M.S. ; Vernon, S.D. & Horvath, S. (2008). Integrated Weighted Gene Co-expression Network Analysis with an Application to Chronic Fatigue Syndrome. *BMC Systems Biology*. Vol.2

Puri, B.K. Long-chain Polyunsaturated Fatty Acids and the Pathophysiology of Myalgic Encephalomyelitis (chronic farigue syndrome). (2007). *Jounral of Clinical Pathology*. Vol.60. pp.122-124

Puri, B.K. ; Holmes, J. & Hamilton, G. (2004) Eicosapentaenoic Acid-rich Essential Fatty Acid Supplementation in Chronic Fatigue Syndrome Associated with Symptom Remission and Structural Brain Changes. *Int. J. Clin. Pract.* Vol.58. pp.297-299

Sanacora, G. ; Gueorguieva, R. ; Epperson, C.N. ; Wu, Y.T., Appel, M. ; Rothman, D.I. ; Krystal, J.H. & Mason, G.F. (2004). Subtype-specific Alterations of Gamma-Aminobutyric Acid and Glutamate in Patients with Major Depression. *Arch. Gen. Psychiatry*. Vol.61. pp.705-713

Schadt, E.E. ; Lamb, J. ; Yang, X. ; Zhu, J. ; Edwards, S. ; GuhaTahkurta, D. ; Sieberts, S.K. ; Monks, S. ; Reitman, M. ; Zhang, C. ; Lum, P.Y. ; Leonardson, A. ; Thieringer, R. ; Metzger, J.M. ; Yang, L. ; Castle, J. ; Zhu, H. ; Kash, S.F. ; Drake, T.A. ; Sachs, A. & Lusis A.J. (2005). An Integrative Genomics Approach to Infer Causal Associations Between Gene Expression and Disease. *Nature Genetics*. Vol.37, No.7, pp.710-717

Schena, M. ; Shalon D. ; Davis, R.W. & Brown P.O. (1995) Quantitative Monitoring of Gene Expression Patterns with a Complementary DNA Microarray. *Science*. Vol.270, No.5235, pp.467-470

Tusher, G. ; Ribshirani, R. & Chu, G. Significance analysis of microarrays applied to the ionizing radiation response. (2001). *Proc. Natl. Acad, Sci.* Vol.98, pp.5116-5121

Van Strater, A.C.P. & Bouby, P.F. (2006). Omega-3 Fatty Acids and Mood Disorders. *Am. J. Psychiatr.* Vol.163. p.2018

Webster, J.I. ; Tonelli, L. & Sternberg, E.M. (2002) Neuroendocrine Regulation of Immunity. *Annu. Rev. Immunol.* Vol.20. pp.125-163

4

Corticosteroid-Binding Globulin Gene Mutations and Chronic Fatigue/Pain Syndromes: An Overview of Current Evidence

C. S. Marathe and D. J. Torpy
The University of Adelaide, Australia

1. Introduction

Several lines of evidence suggest that corticosteroid-binding globulin (CBG), long known as a cortisol-transport glycoprotein, may have broader roles in targeted-tissue hormone delivery and the neurobehavioural responses to stress. These include studies of individual kindreds with rare severe CBG gene (*SERPINA6)* mutations, a study of chronic fatigue patients, a community study of individuals with a relatively high prevalence of two function altering CBG gene mutations in Calabria, Italy, a study of the genetic epidemiology of chronic pain, and, finally, two separate animal CBG gene knockout models.

2. Corticosteroid-binding globulin: Structure and function

CBG circulates as a 383 amino acid (50-55kDa) glycoprotein in blood, and was discovered in the late 1950s[1-6] as a transport glycoprotein for cortisol in human plasma[7,8]. The liver is the main source of circulating CBG, although gene expression is also present in the placenta and kidney, and CBG is differentially expressed according to developmental stage in foetal life[9,10]. CBG is highly glycosylated with six consensus sites for N-glycosylation and sialyation[11]. Each molecule contains a single high-affinity (Ka = 1.7x 10^8) cortisol binding site[12,13], for which glycosylation at Asn^{238} appears to be critical, probably due to the effect of this glycosylation site on tertiary structure[14]. Deglycosylation of the mature protein does not alter cortisol binding affinity. CBG is a Clade A member of the serine protease inhibitor (serpin) superfamily, however it lacks intrinsic serine protease inhibitory activity[15,16]. The CBG (SERPINA6) gene is located in a group of other serine protease inhibitor genes, thought to be phylogenetically related, on chromosome 14q31 - q32.1[17].

Approximately 80% of circulating cortisol under basal conditions is bound to CBG. About 5-8% of the cortisol is in a free or an unfractionated state, which is generally thought to be the biologically active form, and the remainder is loosely bound to high capacity albumin[18]. CBG, as part of its biological function, undergoes a so called 'stressed to relaxed' (S→R) conformational change following the cleavage of its surface-exposed loop called the reactive centre loop or RCL[18]. However, the mode of cleavage in CBG differs from other members of the serpin superfamily[19]. The RCL of CBG is cleaved by human leukocyte elastase (HLE) at sites of inflammation[10,20] rather than by inhibiting proteinases[18]. The HLE cleavage of CBG results in a ten-fold decrease in its binding affinity[21], thus releasing cortisol[10]. In states of stress such as sepsis[22], burns[23] and myocardial infarction[24], the free cortisol percentage increases to up to 20%, due to the saturation of available CBG by increased cortisol and reduced CBG levels (a result of increased CBG cleavage/catabolism and inhibited synthesis)[25,26]. Inflammatory cytokines such as IL-6, glucocorticoids, insulin, hyperthyroidism, nephrotic syndrome, and cirrhosis can also reduce CBG concentrations. On the other hand, oestrogen and pregnancy can increase CBG concentrations[10,27]. It is interesting to note, in this context, that increased production of HLE by neutrophils has been reported in chronic fatigue syndrome[20,28].

3. Corticosteroid-binding globulin: More than just a transport glycoprotein

CBG has traditionally been considered to be a transport vehicle for the water insoluble cortisol[29], with perhaps some role in moderating release of free cortisol in times of cortisol excess or deficiency[30]. This is in keeping with the 'free hormone hypothesis' proposed by Mendel[31], which states that the biological activity of a hormone depends on the free rather than its protein-bound concentrations. The free steroid hormone can cross the plasma membrane of the target cell due to its small size and lipid solubility[32].

However, there is evidence that suggests that CBG-bound cortisol could play a functional role different to unbound cortisol. While a specific CBG cell receptor has not yet been cloned, cell membrane binding sites for CBG, which share many features of a receptor, have been known for some time[33,34]. This has led some to speculate that CBG may act as a hormone and there may be a direct contribution of bound cortisol in glucocorticoid bioavailability via this yet unidentified CBG receptor[34]. Accumulation of cyclic AMP[35] occurs as a result of this CBG:cell receptor interaction. Recently, it has been shown that the NeuAc residues on the N-glycans restrict the binding of CBG to the cell receptor. Removing these NeuAc residues resulted in marked increase in cyclic AMP levels[35]. Dilution of CBG results in release of cortisol and thus suggests, at the very least, an indirect contribution of bound cortisol in glucocorticoid bioavailability[36].

A closely related steroid binding glycoprotein in the human body is sex hormone binding globulin (SHBG), which binds testosterone and oestradiol. A role for SHBG beyond transport has been shown. Sex steroid tissue delivery involves endocytic uptake of SHBG–sex steroid complexes via the LDL receptor–related protein member megalin[37]. Megalin knockout mice exhibit sexual infantilism[37]. While possible a megalin-like mechanism for endocytic uptake of CBG-cortisol complexes has not been demonstrated.

4. Chronic fatigue/pain syndromes, the concept of 'allostasis' and the role of hypothalamo-pituitary-adrenal axis

Chronic fatigue/pain syndromes are common. Epidemiological studies have estimated the point prevalence of chronic widespread pain (CWP) in the community to be up to 11%[38], and about 9% of the total population will experience significant chronic fatigue at any one time[39]. It should be noted, however, that up to two-thirds of these patients complaining of chronic fatigue will not meet the criteria for chronic fatigue syndrome (CFS)[40,41]. A considerable overlap exists, however, in terms of both clinical and biochemical characteristics, and perhaps the pathogenesis of chronic fatigue and chronic pain[42].

CFS is a clinical diagnosis, the hallmark of which is disabling fatigue for over six months with prolonged (>24hrs) post-exertional exacerbation along with other symptoms which include impaired short-term memory and concentration, sore throat, tender lymph nodes, myalgia, arthralgia, headaches and unrefreshing sleep[43]. Since the term 'chronic fatigue syndrome' was proposed in 1988 to replace the prior 'chronic Epstein Barr virus syndrome' (based on the realization that not all chronic fatigue cases were post-infective in nature)[44], newer aetiological models based on neuroendocrine[45], psychiatric[46], evolutionary[47], immunological[48] and non–infective inflammatory[49] mechanisms have been described. A well-accepted explanation for the development of CFS or even the relative contribution of the different possible mechanisms, however, remains elusive. CFS, a debilitating disease sharing many features with fibromyalgia[50], CWP and similar idiopathic chronic fatigue syndromes, significantly impairs a patient's quality of life[51,52], social[53] and emotional well being[54,55], besides putting considerable economic strain on the community[56]. It is, therefore, imperative that a better understanding of the causation of CFS and related disorders is achieved to enable development of effective therapeutic options, which are currently lacking[57].

A hereditary component to CFS has also been suggested[58-60]. Recently, an analysis of the Utah population database (UPDB) looking at the genetic relationships of CFS patients was published[61]. 811 patients diagnosed with CFS by the US CDC or the Fukuda criteria[43] underwent genealogical analysis. A significant excess in CFS relative risk among first (2.70, 95% CI: 1.56-4.66), second (2.34, 95% CI: 1.31-4.19), and third degree relatives (1.93, 95% CI: 1.21-3.07) was observed.

The human stress system includes the two effector arms, the hypothalamic-pituitary-adrenal axis (HPA axis) and the sympathetic nervous system, with their chief hormonal products, cortisol and noradrenaline/adrenaline, respectively. The stress system responds in a highly coordinated and stress-specific manner to stressors, which may be defined as threats to homeostasis or the stable internal milieu of the organism. Stressors such as infection, inflammation, trauma, and psychic disturbance such as fear or anxiety act via inflammatory cytokines or internal CNS influences to produce a range of physiological responses designed to protect the body from stress, such as elevated blood pressure, redirection of blood flow, mobilization of metabolic substrates and CNS arousal. The stress system has basal tone and it has been proposed that altered chronic stress system activity, which may be produced by excessive stress at key developmental stages such as intrauterine, childhood and adolescence, may be detrimental to health. For example, excessive stress system activity may lead to metabolic deterioration such as hypertension, diabetes, central adiposity, osteoporosis and mental illness, which together comprise a high proportion of modern chronic illnesses. Chronically altered stress system activity may be described as a state of allostasis representing stability but with risk of long term tissue damage[62].

On the other hand, reduced stress system activity, another form of allostasis, may be expected to produce a state of hypo-arousal and lack of anti-nociceptive activity centrally, leading to the many chronic pain and fatigue based disorders (CFS, fibromyalgia, irritable bowel syndrome, migraine and many others). A number of studies have shown relative hypocortisolism in pain/fatigue disorders[63-65]. In patients with CFS, studies have demonstrated low levels of cortisol in plasma[63,64] (in morning[63] as well as in the evening[66]), urine[63,67-70] and saliva[70-73]. Corticotropin-releasing hormone (CRH) and adrenocorticotropic hormone (ACTH) challenge tests, which test adequacy of the HPA axis also show similar results in CFS patients[63] although not consistently[45]. Hypocortisolism has also been shown in patients with fibromyalgia[74-76] and chronic pain syndromes[77,78]. Chronic fatigue syndrome has a strikingly high female preponderance (up to 75%) and it has been shown that the glucocorticoid sensitivity of pro-inflammatory cytokine production after psychological stress is different among the sexes[79].

5. CBG gene mutation: Kindred studies

Four major function altering mutations of the CBG gene have been described in humans. These include CBG Leuven, CBG Lyon, CBG null and a CBG non-cortisol binding variant. Old and new genetic nomenclature for these mutations is shown in Table 1. CBG Leuven (c.344T>A, p.Leu115His) reduces CBG:cortisol binding three-fold[15,80]. CBG Lyon has been described in three kindreds and reduces cortisol binding affinity 4-fold (c.1165G>A, p.Asp389Asn)[15,81]. CBG null (c.32G>A, p.Trp11X) prevents CBG synthesis and homozygotes are completely CBG deficient[82]. Both CBG Lyon and null are associated with fatigue and chronic pain and were described together in single kindred where the phenotype was similar[82]. The description of a kindred with a non-cortisol binding variant of CBG included an index case with fatigue[83].

Mutations and polymorphisms	Coding DNA (old nomenclature)	Coding DNA (new nomenclature)	Protein (old nomenclature)	Protein (new nomenclature)
Leuven	T433A	c.344T>A	Leu93His	p.Leu115His
Lyon	G1254A	c.1165G>A	Asp367Asn	p.Asp389Asn
Null	G121A	c.32G>A	Trp-12X	p.Trp11X
Non-cortisol binding	-	c.776G>T	p.Gly237Val	p.Gly259Val
p.Ala246Ser polymorphism	c.825G>T	c.736G>T	Ala-Ser224	p.Ala246Ser

Table 1. Old and new nomenclature for known mutations and polymorphisms in *CBG*

6. CBG null

We have described a 39 member Italian-Australian kindred with a novel null (complete loss-of-function) CBG mutation, an exon 2 mutation causing premature termination codon corresponding to residue-12 (c121G→A)[82] (Fig. 1). The 48 year-old female proband was found to have low total plasma cortisol levels but normal 24-hour urinary free cortisol. She had an elevated plasma cortisol fraction and undetectable CBG levels. CBG gene sequencing of the family revealed two null homozygotes, 19 null heterozygotes, three Lyon heterozygotes and two compound (Null/Lyon) heterozygotes. CBG levels were also undetectable in the other two CBG null homozygotes. There was a 50% CBG reduction in the null heterozygotes and an even greater reduction in the compound heterozygotes. Five members of the family, including the female proband, met the United States' Centre for Disease Control (CDC) criteria[43] for chronic fatigue syndrome. In addition, 12 out of the 14 members with heterozygote mutation and two out of three with homozygous mutation were found to have idiopathic chronic fatigue. Pain syndromes were observed in six subjects with null mutation - four were null heterozygotes while two were homozygotes. One of these pain affected null subjects also fulfilled the criteria for CFS. Prior to finding this family with CBG null deficiency it had been thought that complete CBG deficiency was incompatible with life[9,84].

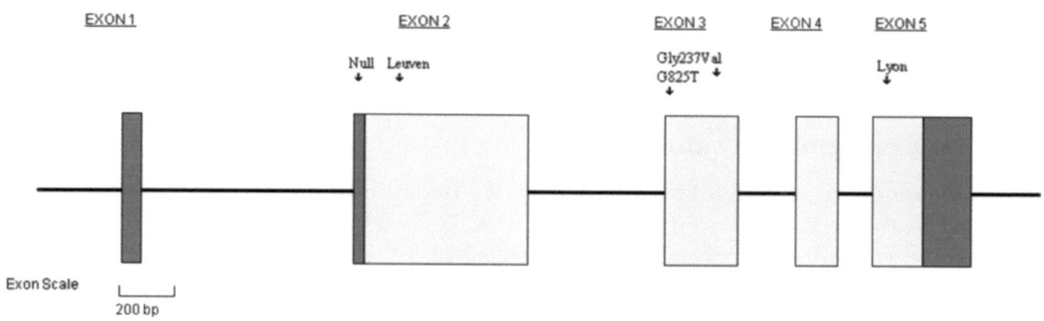

Fig. 1. Schematic diagram of the CBG gene and the location of CBG mutations. Darker shaded portions indicate regions of the exons that are untranslated. The mutations include CBG null (G121A; Trp-12X), transcortin Leuven (T433A; Leu93His), CBG Lyon (G1254A; Asp367Asn) and Ser/Ala224 polymorphism (G825T) and CBG non -binding polymorphism (Gly237Val).

7. CBG Lyon

The CBG variant produced due to a missense mutation, an aspartic acid to aspargine substitution at residue 367 ($Asp^{367} \rightarrow Asn$) was first described in a 43 year old woman of northwest African origin in Lyon, France, and is known as the CBG Lyon mutation[81]. Her main symptoms included chronic asthenia, depressive mood and hypotension. She was found to have very low total plasma cortisol but normal ACTH and urine free cortisol levels. A low free cortisol concentration suggested an abnormality in CBG binding and was later confirmed. Her four children were all found to heterozygous for this mutation.

Since then, CBG Lyon has been described in two other kindreds[82,85]. The mutation has been reported in a 40 year-old white Brazilian woman presenting with chronic fatigue and hypotension. The family members screened, including her parents and her children, were found to be heterozygous for the mutation but did not complain of chronic fatigue[85]. We have also reported CBG Lyon mutation in the family members of a proband with CBG null mutation[82]. Three family members were CBG Lyon heterozygotes, while two had co-inheritance of CBG Lyon and CBG null (compound heterozygotes). The family members with co-inheritance had clearly low CBG levels. All available family members with CBG Lyon mutation, both heterozygotes and compound heterozygotes reported significant fatigue[82].

8. CBG non-binding Gly 237 Val

This CBG gene polymorphism, involving a c.776g>t transversion in exon 3 of the *SERPINA6* gene resulting in a p.Gly237Val substitution, was described recently in a 26 year-old Pakistani–British woman presenting with fatigue and hypotension. This CBG variant lacks any steroid binding activity. Two siblings were found homozygous for this mutation and two more family members (including the proband's mother) were found to be heterozygous. The homozygous members had reduced CBG levels (about 50% for the proband) by RIA measurements but undetectable CBG when measured with cortisol-binding capacity assays. However, aside from the proband, none of the family members, including two siblings found homozygous for the mutation, reported symptoms of chronic pain or fatigue. The only biochemical finding that differentiated the proband from the other homozygous members was the increased cortisol pulsatility[83].

9. Genetic epidemiology studies

Given the evidence from the kindred studies, we hypothesized that CBG polymorphisms could act as a genetic risk factor for patients with CFS. Two hundred and forty eight patients with CFS and an equal number of control subjects had full CBG gene sequencing. An exon 3 polymorphism (c.825G-->T, Ala-Ser224) was more commonly observed in CFS patients than expected by chance at the trend level ($P<0.07$), suggesting that homozygosity for the serine allele of the CBG gene may predispose to CFS[86].

We also conducted a population-based study in Calabria, Italy, the region our Italian-Australian null/Lyon kindred originated from, to look at the prevalence of CBG mutations in the local community. The results showed a high prevalence of CBG null and Lyon mutations (3.6%). Chronic widespread pain, but not chronic fatigue, was found to be common in subjects with CBG mutation[87].

Genetic influences have been postulated to account for 50% of the variance as well as the reduced pain thresholds seen in chronic pain syndromes[88,89]. The prospective population-based cohort study EPIFUND (Epidemiology of functional disorders), examined if genetic variation within the HPA axis genes was associated with susceptibility to musculoskeletal pain. The CBG gene (SERPINA6) and six other HPA axis genes CRH, CRH receptor 1 (CRHR1), CRH binding protein (CRHBP), the ACTH precursor pro-opiomelanocortin (POMC) and its receptor (MC2R), the glucocorticoid receptor (NR3C1) were examined. Seventy-five single nucleotide polymorphisms (SNPs) were detected in 164 CWP patients and 172 pain-free controls. Amongst the seven HPA axis genes, the most notable genetic variation was in the *SERPINA6* gene. Two SNPs in *SERPINA6* (rs 941601 and rs 8022616), located within a single haplotype block, were significantly associated with CWP. Moreover, in patients reporting pain, four SNPs of *SERPINA6* were associated with the maximum number of pain sites[88]. This finding assumes significance given that there was no association with SNPs in CRH, CRHR1, CRHBP, POMC or NR3C1 and CWP was observed and only a single SNP in MC2R, rs11661134, was associated with increased odds of having CWP.

CBG gene knockout mice models

The effect of a gene deletion can also be studied in the laboratory setting by producing 'knockout gene' mouse models, achieved by a homologous recombination between DNA sequences in the existing chromosome and the newly introduced DNA into pluripotent embryo-derived stem cells[90]. In the study reported by Richard et al, the CBG gene knockout mouse was created by 'floxing' - contraction for flanking the lox p sites - exon 2 of the *SERPINA6* gene[91]. The learned helplessness paradigm[92], an animal model of depression, was used to evaluate behavioural changes following intense stress. HPA axis dysregulation has previously been linked to helpless behavior[93,94]. The CBG deficient mice (Cbg -/-) showed increased immobility in the forced-swimming test and markedly enhanced learned helplessness after prolonged uncontrollable stress (footshock) as well as markedly reduced total circulating corticosterone in both rested and stressed states. Responses to milder stressors was not altered. In another CBG knockout mice study[95], Cbg -/- mice had a reduction in CBG levels and a correspondingly ten-fold increase in levels of free cortisol. Despite this, there was no evidence of enhanced glucocorticoid activity, suggesting the role of CBG in mediating corticosteroid functions. More importantly, Cbg -/- mice exhibited a possible fatigue syndrome, characterised by reduced activity levels compared with the control group. The elevated cortisol and reduced activity levels were not seen in the study of Richard et al[91]. Taken together, however, these findings suggest an important hitherto unanticipated role for CBG in the neurobehavioural aspects of stress system function.

10. Conclusion

There is an unequivocal role for CBG as a transport molecule for cortisol, and altered levels of CBG are generally met with unaltered levels of free cortisol, confirming it is free cortisol which is actively regulated in blood.

However, recent studies have linked rare CBG gene mutations, which alter CBG levels or binding affinity, to pain/fatigue syndromes. This association is not universal suggesting that other genetic or environmental factors influence the phenotype. Genetic epidemiology studies point to the CBG gene and its variants as having a role in the risk of developing a chronic pain phenotype. Animal studies have also shown that CBG genetic deletions can produce altered neurobehavioural responses to stress. This mounting evidence suggests a role for CBG in tissue delivery or other elements of stress system function, although the precise mechanisms await elucidation.

11. Acknowledgement

The authors would like to thanks Dr B Ardesjö Lundgren for her expertise in preparing Table 1.

12. References

[1] Daughaday WH. Binding of corticosteroids by plasma proteins. II. Paper electrophoresis and equilibrium paper electrophoresis. *J Clin Invest.* Dec 1956;35(12):1434-1438.
[2] Daughaday WH. Binding of corticosteroids by plasma proteins. I. Dialysis equilibrium and renal clearance studies. *J Clin Invest.* Dec 1956;35(12):1428-1433.
[3] Daughaday WH. Binding of corticosteroids by plasma proteins. IV. The electrophoretic demonstration of corticosteroid binding globulin. *J Clin Invest.* Apr 1958;37(4):519-523.
[4] Daughaday WH. Binding of corticosteroids by plasma proteins. III. The binding of corticosteroid and related hormones by human plasma and plasma protein fractions as measured by equilibrium dialysis. *J Clin Invest.* Apr 1958;37(4):511-518.

[5] Daughaday WH. Binding of corticosteroids by plasma proteins. V. Corticosteroid-binding globulin activity in normal human beings and in certain disease states. *AMA Arch Intern Med.* Feb 1958;101(2):286-290.

[6] Sandberg AA, Slaunwhite WR, Jr., Antoniades HN. The binding of steroids and steroid conjugates to human plasma proteins. *Recent Prog Horm Res.* 1957;13:209-260; discussion 260-207.

[7] Brien TG. Human corticosteroid binding globulin. *Clin Endocrinol (Oxf).* Feb 1981;14(2):193-212.

[8] Ghose-Dastidar J, Ross JB, Green R. Expression of biologically active human corticosteroid binding globulin by insect cells: acquisition of function requires glycosylation and transport. *Proc Natl Acad Sci U S A.* Aug 1 1991;88(15):6408-6412.

[9] Challis JR, Berdusco ET, Jeffray TM, Yang K, Hammond GL. Corticosteroid-binding globulin (CBG) in fetal development. *J Steroid Biochem Mol Biol.* Jun 1995;53(1-6):523-527.

[10] Hammond GL, Smith CL, Underhill CM, Nguyen VT. Interaction between corticosteroid binding globulin and activated leukocytes in vitro. *Biochem Biophys Res Commun.* Oct 15 1990;172(1):172-177.

[11] Hammond GL, Smith CL, Goping IS, et al. Primary structure of human corticosteroid binding globulin, deduced from hepatic and pulmonary cDNAs, exhibits homology with serine protease inhibitors. *Proc Natl Acad Sci U S A.* Aug 1987;84(15):5153-5157.

[12] Kojima N, Sakata S, Komaki T, Matsuda M, Miura K. [Preparation of an immunoadsorbent interacting specifically with cortisol-binding globulin (CBG) and its application to the interaction between CBG and cortisol--evaluation of the association constant (Ka) between CBG and cortisol in normal subjects]. *Nippon Naibunpi Gakkai Zasshi.* May 20 1987;63(5):695-701.

[13] Hammond GL, Smith CL, Underhill DA. Molecular studies of corticosteroid binding globulin structure, biosynthesis and function. *J Steroid Biochem Mol Biol.* 1991;40(4-6):755-762.

[14] Avvakumov GV, Warmels-Rodenhiser S, Hammond GL. Glycosylation of human corticosteroid-binding globulin at aspargine 238 is necessary for steroid binding. *J Biol Chem.* Jan 15 1993;268(2):862-866.

[15] Gagliardi L, Ho JT, Torpy DJ. Corticosteroid-binding globulin: the clinical significance of altered levels and heritable mutations. *Mol Cell Endocrinol.* Mar 5 2010;316(1):24-34.

[16] Klieber MA, Underhill C, Hammond GL, Muller YA. Corticosteroid-binding globulin, a structural basis for steroid transport and proteinase-triggered release. *J Biol Chem.* Oct 5 2007;282(40):29594-29603.

[17] Seralini GE, Berube D, Gagne R, Hammond GL. The human corticosteroid binding globulin gene is located on chromosome 14q31-q32.1 near two other serine protease inhibitor genes. *Hum Genet.* Nov 1990;86(1):73-75.

[18] Gettins PG. Serpin structure, mechanism, and function. *Chem Rev.* Dec 2002;102(12):4751-4804.

[19] Qi X, Loiseau F, Chan WL, et al. Allosteric modulation of hormone release from thyroxine and corticosteroid-binding globulins. *J Biol Chem.* May 6 2011;286(18):16163-16173.

[20] Pemberton PA, Stein PE, Pepys MB, Potter JM, Carrell RW. Hormone binding globulins undergo serpin conformational change in inflammation. *Nature.* Nov 17 1988;336(6196):257-258.

[21] Zhou A, Wei Z, Stanley PL, Read RJ, Stein PE, Carrell RW. The S-to-R transition of corticosteroid-binding globulin and the mechanism of hormone release. *J Mol Biol.* Jun 27 2008;380(1):244-251.

[22] Pugeat M, Bonneton A, Perrot D, et al. Decreased immunoreactivity and binding activity of corticosteroid-binding globulin in serum in septic shock. *Clin Chem.* Aug 1989;35(8):1675-1679.

[23] Bernier J, Jobin N, Emptoz-Bonneton A, Pugeat MM, Garrel DR. Decreased corticosteroid-binding globulin in burn patients: relationship with interleukin-6 and fat in nutritional support. *Crit Care Med.* Mar 1998;26(3):452-460.

[24] Zouaghi H, Savu L, Guerot C, Gryman R, Coulon A, Nunez EA. Total and unbound cortisol-, progesterone-, oestrone- and transcortin-binding activities in sera from patients with myocardial infarction: evidence for differential responses of good and bad prognostic cases. *Eur J Clin Invest.* Dec 1985;15(6):365-370.

[25] Ho JT, Al-Musalhi H, Chapman MJ, et al. Septic shock and sepsis: a comparison of total and free plasma cortisol levels. *J Clin Endocrinol Metab.* Jan 2006;91(1):105-114.

[26] Papanicolaou DA, Wilder RL, Manolagas SC, Chrousos GP. The pathophysiologic roles of interleukin-6 in human disease. *Ann Intern Med.* Jan 15 1998;128(2):127-137.

[27] Stewart PM, Clark PM. The low-dose corticotropin-stimulation test revisited: the less, the better? *Nat Clin Pract Endocrinol Metab.* Feb 2009;5(2):68-69.

[28] Demettre E, Bastide L, D'Haese A, et al. Ribonuclease L proteolysis in peripheral blood mononuclear cells of chronic fatigue syndrome patients. *J Biol Chem.* Sep 20 2002;277(38):35746-35751.

[29] Dunn JF, Nisula BC, Rodbard D. Transport of steroid hormones: binding of 21 endogenous steroids to both testosterone-binding globulin and corticosteroid-binding globulin in human plasma. *J Clin Endocrinol Metab.* Jul 1981;53(1):58-68.

[30] Torpy DJ, Ho JT. Corticosteroid-binding globulin gene polymorphisms: clinical implications and links to idiopathic chronic fatigue disorders. *Clin Endocrinol (Oxf).* Aug 2007;67(2):161-167.

[31] Mendel CM. The free hormone hypothesis: a physiologically based mathematical model. *Endocr Rev.* Aug 1989;10(3):232-274.

[32] Adams JS. "Bound" to work: the free hormone hypothesis revisited. *Cell.* Sep 9 2005;122(5):647-649.

[33] Nakhla AM, Khan MS, Rosner W. Induction of adenylate cyclase in a mammary carcinoma cell line by human corticosteroid-binding globulin. *Biochem Biophys Res Commun.* Jun 30 1988;153(3):1012-1018.

[34] Rosner W, Hryb DJ, Khan MS, Singer CJ, Nakhla AM. Are corticosteroid-binding globulin and sex hormone-binding globulin hormones? *Ann N Y Acad Sci.* 1988; 538:137-145.

[35] Sumer-Bayraktar Z, Kolarich D, Campbell MP, Ali S, Packer NH, Thaysen-Andersen M. N-glycans modulate the function of human corticosteroid-binding globulin. *Mol Cell Proteomics.* May 10 2011.

[36] Perogamvros I, Kayahara M, Trainer PJ, Ray DW. Serum regulates cortisol bioactivity by corticosteroid-binding globulin dependent and independent mechanisms, as revealed by combined bioassay and physicochemical assay approaches. *Clin Endocrinol (Oxf).* Feb 21 2011.

[37] Hammes A, Andreassen TK, Spoelgen R, et al. Role of endocytosis in cellular uptake of sex steroids. *Cell.* Sep 9 2005;122(5):751-762.

[38] Croft P, Rigby AS, Boswell R, Schollum J, Silman A. The prevalence of chronic widespread pain in the general population. *J Rheumatol.* Apr 1993;20(4):710-713.

[39] Skapinakis P, Lewis G, Meltzer H. Clarifying the relationship between unexplained chronic fatigue and psychiatric morbidity: results from a community survey in Great Britain. *Am J Psychiatry.* Sep 2000;157(9):1492-1498.

[40] Darbishire L, Ridsdale L, Seed PT. Distinguishing patients with chronic fatigue from those with chronic fatigue syndrome: a diagnostic study in UK primary care. *Br J Gen Pract.* Jun 2003;53(491):441-445.

[41] Ridsdale L, Godfrey E, Chalder T, et al. Chronic fatigue in general practice: is counselling as good as cognitive behaviour therapy? A UK randomised trial. *Br J Gen Pract.* Jan 2001;51(462):19-24.

[42] Clauw DJ, Chrousos GP. Chronic pain and fatigue syndromes: overlapping clinical and neuroendocrine features and potential pathogenic mechanisms. *Neuro--immunomodulation.* May-Jun 1997;4(3):134-153.

[43] Fukuda K, Straus SE, Hickie I, Sharpe MC, Dobbins JG, Komaroff A. The chronic fatigue syndrome: a comprehensive approach to its definition and study. International Chronic Fatigue Syndrome Study Group. *Ann Intern Med.* Dec 15 1994;121(12):953-959.

[44] Holmes GP, Kaplan JE, Gantz NM, et al. Chronic fatigue syndrome: a working case definition. *Ann Intern Med.* Mar 1988;108(3):387-389.

[45] Cleare AJ. The neuroendocrinology of chronic fatigue syndrome. *Endocr Rev.* Apr 2003;24(2):236-252.

[46] Byrne E. Idiopathic chronic fatigue and myalgia syndrome (myalgic encephalomyelitis): some thoughts on nomenclature and aetiology. *Med J Aust.* Jan 18 1988;148(2):80-82.

[47] Chrousos GP, Kino T. Glucocorticoid signaling in the cell. Expanding clinical implications to complex human behavioral and somatic disorders. *Ann N Y Acad Sci.* Oct 2009;1179:153-166.

[48] Lorusso L, Mikhaylova SV, Capelli E, Ferrari D, Ngonga GK, Ricevuti G. Immunological aspects of chronic fatigue syndrome. *Autoimmun Rev.* Feb 2009;8(4):287-291.

[49] Arnett SV, Alleva LM, Korossy-Horwood R, Clark IA. Chronic fatigue syndrome - A neuroimmunological model. *Med Hypotheses.* Jul 2011;77(1):77-83.

[50] Roitman A, Bruchis S, Bauman B, Kaufman H, Laron Z. Total deficiency of corticosteroid-binding globulin. *Clin Endocrinol (Oxf).* Nov 1984;21(5):541-548.

[51] Schweitzer R, Kelly B, Foran A, Terry D, Whiting J. Quality of life in chronic fatigue syndrome. *Soc Sci Med.* Nov 1995;41(10):1367-1372.

[52] Anderson JS, Ferrans CE. The quality of life of persons with chronic fatigue syndrome. *J Nerv Ment Dis.* Jun 1997;185(6):359-367.

[53] Solomon L, Nisenbaum R, Reyes M, Papanicolaou DA, Reeves WC. Functional status of persons with chronic fatigue syndrome in the Wichita, Kansas, population. *Health Qual Life Outcomes.* 2003;1:48.

[54] Prins JB, van der Meer JW, Bleijenberg G. Chronic fatigue syndrome. *Lancet.* Jan 28 2006;367(9507):346-355.

[55] Wessely S. The epidemiology of chronic fatigue syndrome. *Epidemiol Psichiatr Soc.* Jan-Apr 1998;7(1):10-24.

[56] Reynolds KJ, Vernon SD, Bouchery E, Reeves WC. The economic impact of chronic fatigue syndrome. *Cost Eff Resour Alloc.* Jun 21 2004;2(1):4.

[57] Cairns R, Hotopf M. A systematic review describing the prognosis of chronic fatigue syndrome. *Occup Med (Lond).* Jan 2005;55(1):20-31.

[58] Kaiser J. Biomedicine. Genes and chronic fatigue: how strong is the evidence? *Science.* May 5 2006;312(5774):669-671.

[59] Walsh CM, Zainal NZ, Middleton SJ, Paykel ES. A family history study of chronic fatigue syndrome. *Psychiatr Genet.* Sep 2001;11(3):123-128.
[60] Buchwald D, Herrell R, Ashton S, et al. A twin study of chronic fatigue. *Psychosom Med.* Nov-Dec 2001;63(6):936-943.
[61] Albright F, Light K, Light A, Bateman L, Cannon-Albright LA. Evidence for a heritable predisposition to Chronic Fatigue Syndrome. *BMC Neurol.* 2011;11:62.
[62] Chrousos GP. Stress and disorders of the stress system. *Nat Rev Endocrinol.* Jul 2009;5(7):374-381.
[63] Demitrack MA, Dale JK, Straus SE, et al. Evidence for impaired activation of the hypothalamic-pituitary-adrenal axis in patients with chronic fatigue syndrome. *J Clin Endocrinol Metab.* Dec 1991;73(6):1224-1234.
[64] Poteliakhoff A. Adrenocortical activity and some clinical findings in acute and chronic fatigue. *J Psychosom Res.* 1981;25(2):91-95.
[65] Heim C, Ehlert U, Hellhammer DH. The potential role of hypocortisolism in the pathophysiology of stress-related bodily disorders. *Psychoneuroendocrinology.* Jan 2000;25(1):1-35.
[66] Altemus M, Dale JK, Michelson D, Demitrack MA, Gold PW, Straus SE. Abnormalities in response to vasopressin infusion in chronic fatigue syndrome. *Psychoneuroendocrinology.* Feb 2001;26(2):175-188.
[67] Cleare AJ, Miell J, Heap E, et al. Hypothalamo-pituitary-adrenal axis dysfunction in chronic fatigue syndrome, and the effects of low-dose hydrocortisone therapy. *J Clin Endocrinol Metab.* Aug 2001;86(8):3545-3554.
[68] Hamilos DL, Nutter D, Gershtenson J, et al. Core body temperature is normal in chronic fatigue syndrome. *Biol Psychiatry.* Feb 15 1998;43(4):293-302.
[69] Scott LV, Dinan TG. Urinary free cortisol excretion in chronic fatigue syndrome, major depression and in healthy volunteers. *J Affect Disord.* Jan 1998;47(1-3):49-54.
[70] Young AH, Sharpe M, Clements A, Dowling B, Hawton KE, Cowen PJ. Basal activity of the hypothalamic-pituitary-adrenal axis in patients with the chronic fatigue syndrome (neurasthenia). *Biol Psychiatry.* Feb 1 1998;43(3):236-237.
[71] Gaab J, Huster D, Peisen R, et al. Low-dose dexamethasone suppression test in chronic fatigue syndrome and health. *Psychosom Med.* Mar-Apr 2002;64(2):311-318.
[72] Strickland P, Morriss R, Wearden A, Deakin B. A comparison of salivary cortisol in chronic fatigue syndrome, community depression and healthy controls. *J Affect Disord.* Jan 1998;47(1-3):191-194.
[73] Wood B, Wessely S, Papadopoulos A, Poon L, Checkley S. Salivary cortisol profiles in chronic fatigue syndrome. *Neuropsychobiology.* 1998;37(1):1-4.
[74] Crofford LJ, Pillemer SR, Kalogeras KT, et al. Hypothalamic-pituitary-adrenal axis perturbations in patients with fibromyalgia. *Arthritis Rheum.* Nov 1994;37(11):1583-1592.
[75] Griep EN, Boersma JW, Lentjes EG, Prins AP, van der Korst JK, de Kloet ER. Function of the hypothalamic-pituitary-adrenal axis in patients with fibromyalgia and low back pain. *J Rheumatol.* Jul 1998;25(7):1374-1381.
[76] McCain GA, Tilbe KS. Diurnal hormone variation in fibromyalgia syndrome: a comparison with rheumatoid arthritis. *J Rheumatol Suppl.* Nov 1989;19:154-157.
[77] Elwan O, Abdella M, el Bayad AB, Hamdy S. Hormonal changes in headache patients. *J Neurol Sci.* Nov 1991;106(1):75-81.
[78] Johansson F. Differences in serum cortisol concentrations in organic and psychogenic chronic pain syndromes. *J Psychosom Res.* 1982;26(3):351-358.

[79] Rohleder N, Schommer NC, Hellhammer DH, Engel R, Kirschbaum C. Sex differences in glucocorticoid sensitivity of proinflammatory cytokine production after psychosocial stress. *Psychosom Med.* Nov-Dec 2001;63(6):966-972.

[80] Van Baelen H, Brepoels R, De Moor P. Transcortin Leuven: a variant of human corticosteroid-binding globulin with decreased cortisol-binding affinity. *J Biol Chem.* Apr 10 1982;257(7):3397-3400.

[81] Emptoz-Bonneton A, Cousin P, Seguchi K, et al. Novel human corticosteroid-binding globulin variant with low cortisol-binding affinity. *J Clin Endocrinol Metab.* Jan 2000;85(1):361-367.

[82] Torpy DJ, Bachmann AW, Grice JE, et al. Familial corticosteroid-binding globulin deficiency due to a novel null mutation: association with fatigue and relative hypotension. *J Clin Endocrinol Metab.* Aug 2001;86(8):3692-3700.

[83] Perogamvros I, Underhill C, Henley DE, et al. Novel corticosteroid-binding globulin variant that lacks steroid binding activity. *J Clin Endocrinol Metab.* Oct 2010;95(10): E142-150.

[84] Hammond GL. Molecular properties of corticosteroid binding globulin and the sex-steroid binding proteins. *Endocr Rev.* Feb 1990;11(1):65-79.

[85] Brunner E, Baima J, Vieira TC, Vieira JG, Abucham J. Hereditary corticosteroid-binding globulin deficiency due to a missense mutation (Asp367Asn, CBG Lyon) in a Brazilian kindred. *Clin Endocrinol (Oxf).* Jun 2003;58(6):756-762.

[86] Torpy DJ, Bachmann AW, Gartside M, et al. Association between chronic fatigue syndrome and the corticosteroid-binding globulin gene ALA SER224 polymorphism. *Endocr Res.* Aug 2004;30(3):417-429.

[87] Cizza G BL, Smirne N, Maletta R, Tomaino C, Costanzo A, Gallo M, Lewis JG, Geracitano S, Grassod MB, Potenza G, Monteleone C, Brancati G, Ho JT, Torpy DJ, Bruni AC. Clinical manifestations of highly prevalent corticosteroid binding globulin mutations in a village in southern italy. *J Clin Endocrinol Metab.* 2011.

[88] Holliday KL, Nicholl BI, Macfarlane GJ, Thomson W, Davies KA, McBeth J. Genetic variation in the hypothalamic-pituitary-adrenal stress axis influences susceptibility to musculoskeletal pain: results from the EPIFUND study. *Ann Rheum Dis.* Mar 2010;69(3):556-560.

[89] Kato K, Sullivan PF, Evengard B, Pedersen NL. Importance of genetic influences on chronic widespread pain. *Arthritis Rheum.* May 2006;54(5):1682-1686.

[90] Capecchi MR. The new mouse genetics: altering the genome by gene targeting. *Trends Genet.* Mar 1989;5(3):70-76.

[91] Richard EM, Helbling JC, Tridon C, et al. Plasma transcortin influences endocrine and behavioral stress responses in mice. *Endocrinology.* Feb 2010;151(2):649-659.

[92] Overmier JB, Seligman ME. Effects of inescapable shock upon subsequent escape and avoidance responding. *J Comp Physiol Psychol.* Feb 1967;63(1):28-33.

[93] Henn FA, Vollmayr B. Stress models of depression: forming genetically vulnerable strains. *Neurosci Biobehav Rev.* 2005;29(4-5):799-804.

[94] Papolos DF. Switching, cycling, and antidepressant-induced effects on cycle frequency and course of illness in adult bipolar disorder: a brief review and commentary. *J Child Adolesc Psychopharmacol.* Summer 2003;13(2):165-171.

[95] Petersen HH, Andreassen TK, Breiderhoff T, et al. Hyporesponsiveness to glucocorticoids in mice genetically deficient for the corticosteroid binding globulin. *Mol Cell Biol.* Oct 2006;26(19):7236-7245.

5

Small Heart as a Constitutive Factor Predisposing to Chronic Fatigue Syndrome

Kunihisa Miwa
Miwa Naika Clinic, Toyama, Japan

1. Introduction

The chronic fatigue syndrome (CFS), which affects many young people in modern, stressful society, is an important health problem, characterized by persistent and relapsing, severe disabling fatigue, not resolved by rest, causing a marked reduction of working activity. [1-4] Despite the public health burden imposed by CFS, effective diagnostic, treatment and prevention strategies are not available because the etiology, risk factors and pathophysiology remain unclarified. Various factors have been implicated in the genesis of CFS, including abnormal immune activation, chronic viral infection, impairment of central nervous system, exaggerated oxidative stress and current emotional disorders.[1-8] Diagnosis of CFS can be made only after alternative known medical and psychiatric causes of chronic fatiguing illness have been excluded.[1,3]

2. Chronic Fatigue Syndrome (CFS) and cardiac dysfunction or low cardiac output

Cardiovascular dysfunction such as chronic heart failure, can be a main cause of disabling chronic fatigue and many symptoms seen in CFS patients are common in patients with low cardiac output syndrome. Indeed, accumulating evidence points to a possible problem with circulation in CFS. [9-14] The reported findings included autonomic dysfunction,[15,16] lower plasma volume and/or red cell mass,[17,18] and abnormalities in neurohumoral systems of circulatory control.[19,20] In 2003 Peckerman et al.[10] provided a preliminary indication of reduced cardiac output in patients with severe CFS.

2.1 Small heart syndrome

The concept that a heart small in relation to the body is inadequate for work was first stated by Laennec[21] in 1826. Later Master[22] reported several, so-called "neurocirculatory asthenia" cases with weakness or fatigue even after ordinary exertion, tachycardia, palpitation and dyspnea, who had a small heart shadow on chest radiography. The most frequent complaints are fatigue or weakness, rapid heart, precordial or chest pain, shortness of breath, nervousness, trembling, sweating and fainting, many of them resembling those in CFS patients. Master hypothesized that these symptoms were caused by diminished venous return, diminished cardiac output, anoxemic heart muscle and decreased oxygen saturation of the blood due to congenital or constitutionally small heart. Similarly DaCosta[23] described "irritable heart" in 1871, a peculiar form of functional disorder of the heart seen in the military population during the American Civil War. The disorder frequently presented either after an episode of diarrhea and persisted after the digestive disturbances had diminished, or originated suddenly without previous digestive disorder. Fatigue was an almost universal complaint in DaCosta's syndrome, although symptoms includes palpitation, cardiac pain, headache, dimness of vision and giddiness.[23,24] Diarrhea may lead to dehydration and reduce venous return or preload, resulting in further decreases in stroke volume and cardiac output in subjects with small heart.

The apparent heart size or cardiothoracic ratio (CTR) is influenced by the position of the heart in the thoracic cage. A small heart may be due to a standing or dropped heart resulting from a low diaphragm and a narrow chest in association with a thin physique and low fat content in epicardial and pericardial spaces. Consequently, the pathognomonic significance of small heart has not been established and is now being overlooked or even ignored.[25]

In order to clarify the pathophysiological significance of small heart syndrome as a cardiovascular disease, we studied 47 patients (16 men and 31 women, mean age: 29±6 years) with a small heart shadow (CTR ≤42% on a chest roentgenogram) and without significant systemic disease who consecutively visited our clinic with possible cardiovascular symptoms, as well as 24 controls (C). These patients with small heart syndrome were divided into 2 groups, 25 patients with severe symptoms (S) and 22 patients with mild ones (M), according to the presence or absence of cardiovascular symptoms including general malaise, easy fatigability, fainting, dizziness, weakness, chest pain, dyspnea and palpitations that were sufficiently severe to significantly disturb their occupational, educational, social or personal activities. Figures 1 and 2 show the chest X roentgenograms of typical cases of group S.

All individuals underwent standard M-mode and two-dimensional echocardiography. The left ventricular (LV) dimensions were measured according to the recommendations of the American Society of Echocardiography.[26] LV volume was calculated by the Teichholz' formura,[27] and an ejection feaction was obtained by the conventional method.

Results are summarized in Tables 1 and 2 and Figures 3-6. As shown in Table 1, the symptom of general malaise and/or easy fatigability was significantly more frequent in S than in M (88% vs. 50%, $p<0.05$). In addition, symptoms including orthostatic dizziness, shortness of breath, dyspnea on effort, palpitations, fainting and chest pain were more frequent in S than in M, although no significant difference was found. In addition, physical findings including narrow chest, foot coldness, pretibial pitting edema, bimanual right kidney palpability, epigastric splash sound, mid-systolic click, late systolic murmur and hypotension were more frequently noted in S than in M, although no significant difference was found.

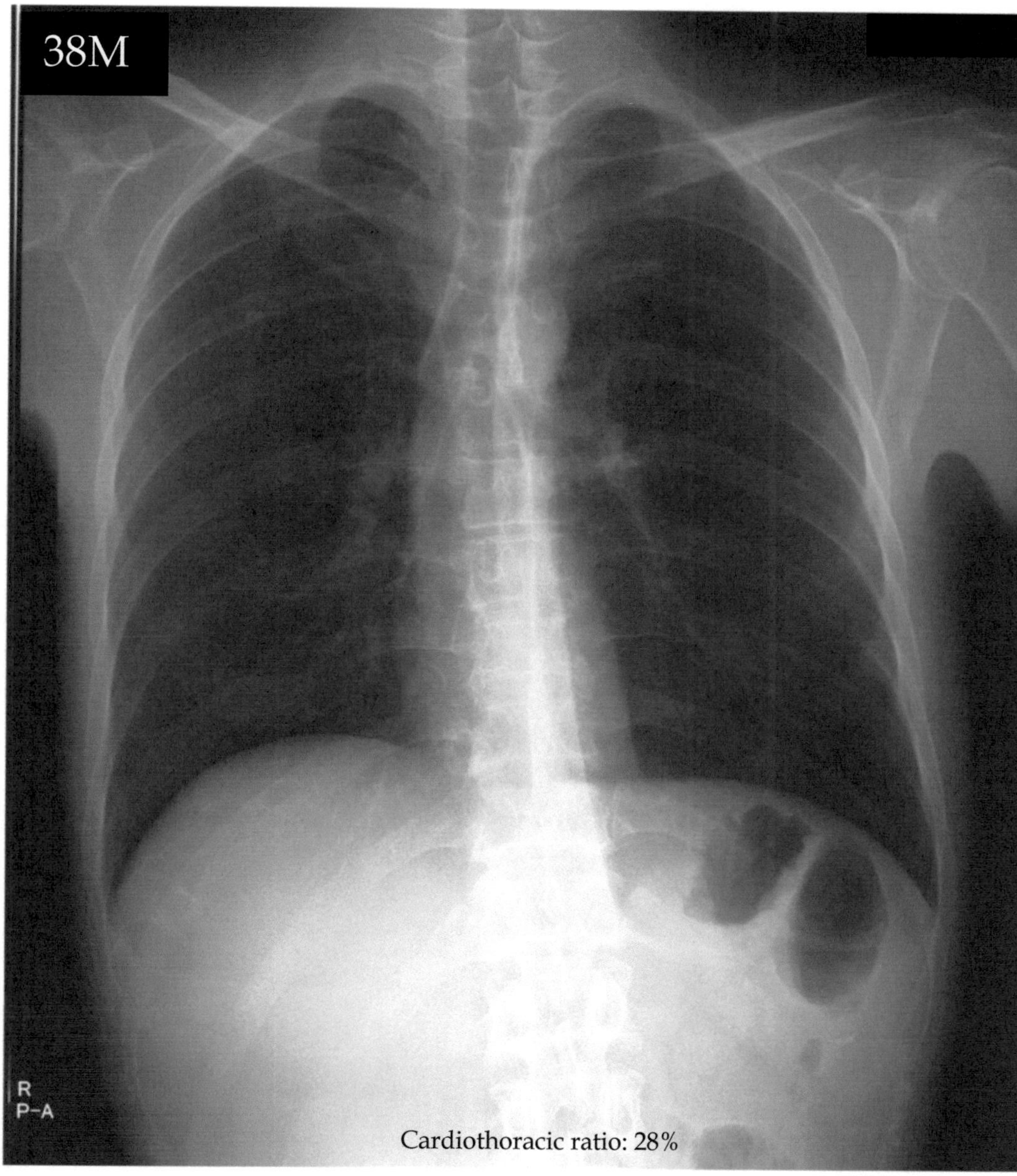

Fig. 1. Chest roentgenogram of a 38-year-old male patient with small heart syndrome (cardiothoracic ratio: 28%) in which vertebral scoliosis was also noted. From about 15 years ago, the patient suffered from severe general malaise, easy fatigability, dyspnea on effort, palpitations and chest pain. He also occasionally developed severe dyspnea with hyperventilation, trembling, sweating and sleep disturbance. He found that upon obtaining employment, he could not work as expected. Upon consulting a psychiatrist 10 years ago, he was diagnosed with anxiety neurosis and treated with medication. He subsequently developed alcoholism. He frequently visited emergency outclinics due to severe dyspnea and anxiety.

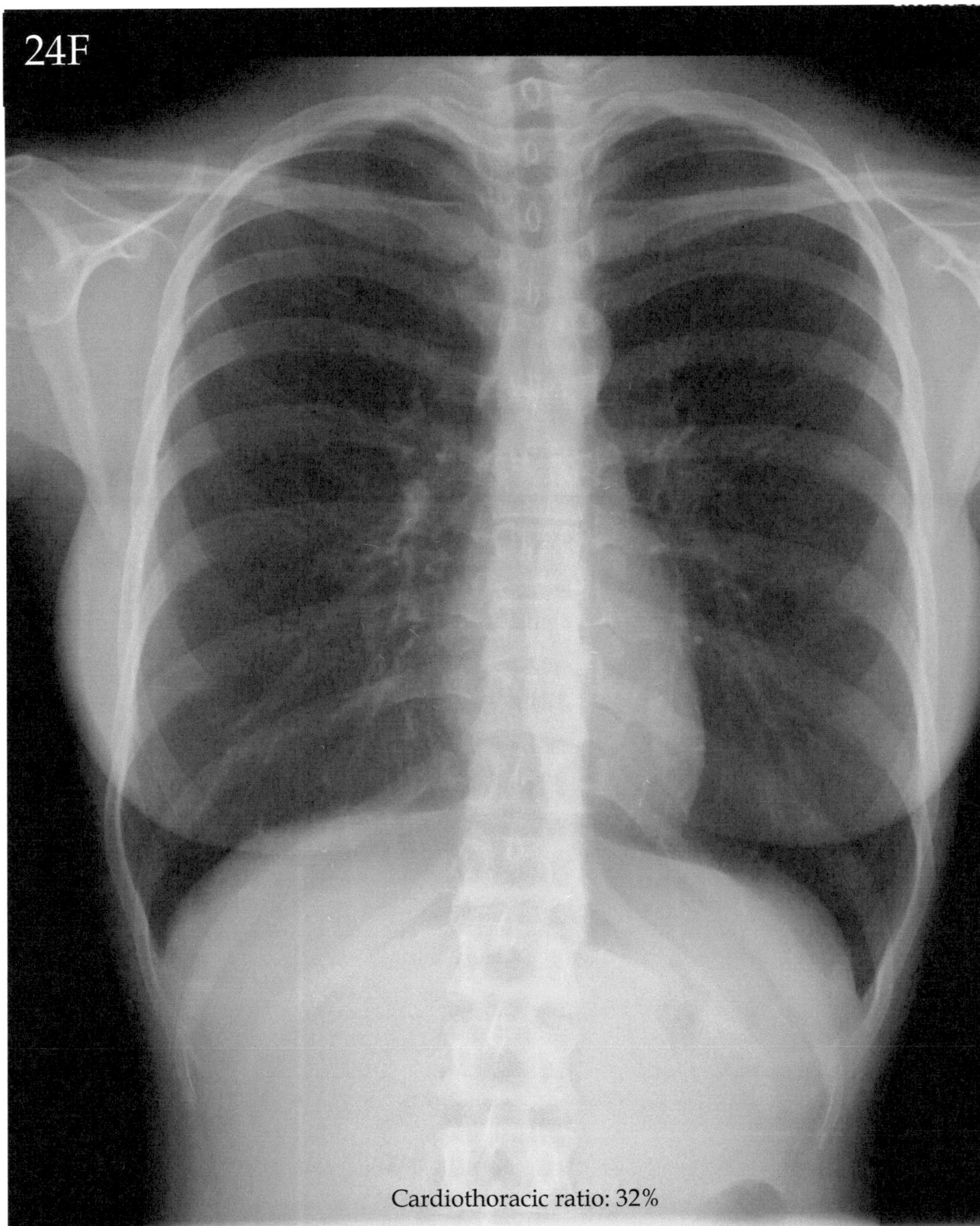

Fig. 2. Chest roentgenogram of a 24-year-old female patient with small heart syndrome (cardiothoracic ratio: 32%). For about 7 years, the patient suffered from severe general fatigue, fainting and orthostatic dizziness. She also frequently developed a headache, chest pain and a sore throat. She was frequently unable to work as a dietician due to increasingly impaired short-term memory and concentration.

	Small heart syndrome		
	Mild (M)	p value	Severe (S)
Number of patients	22		25
Sex (male/female)	7/15		8/17
Age (years)	30±7	NS	28±6
Symptoms			
General malaise	10 (45%)	NS	18 (72%)
Easy fatigability	7 (32%)	NS	14 (56%)
General malaise and/or easy fatigability	11 (50%)	<0.05	22 (88%)
Orthostatic dizziness	8 (36%)	NS	11 (44%)
Shortness of breath	4 (18%)	NS	7 (28%)
Dyspnea on effort	5 (23%)	NS	9 (36%)
Palpitations	5 (23%)	NS	7 (28%)
Faintng	5 (23%)	NS	9 (36%)
Chest pain	7 (32%)	NS	10 (40%)
Physical findings			
Narrow chest	11 (50%)	NS	18 (72%)
Foot coldness	8 (36%)	NS	16 (64%)
Pretibial pitting edema	5 (23%)	NS	9 (36%)
Right kidney palpability	9 (41%)	NS	14 (56%)
Epigastric splash sound	3 (14%)	NS	6 (24%)
Mid-systolic click	2 (9%)	NS	3 (12%)
Late systolic murmur	4 (18%)	NS	5 (20%)
Hypotension (SBP <100 mmHg)	5 (23%)	NS	8 (32%)

M: patients with small heart syndrome and mild symptoms, S: patients with small heart syndrome and severe symptoms, NS: not significant, SBP: systolic blood pressure

Table 1. Comparison of the prevalence of symptoms and physical findings between the study groups with mild or severe symptoms

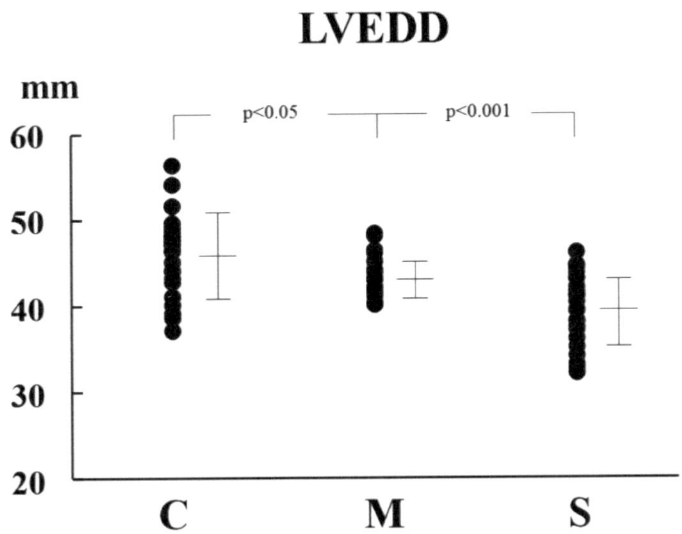

Fig. 3. Comparison of the left ventricular end-diastolic dimension (LVEDD) among the study groups. The mean LVEDD was significantly smaller in S (patients with small heart syndrome and severe symptoms) than in M (patients with small heart syndrome and mild symptoms) and C (control subjects). It was also significantly smaller in M than in C.

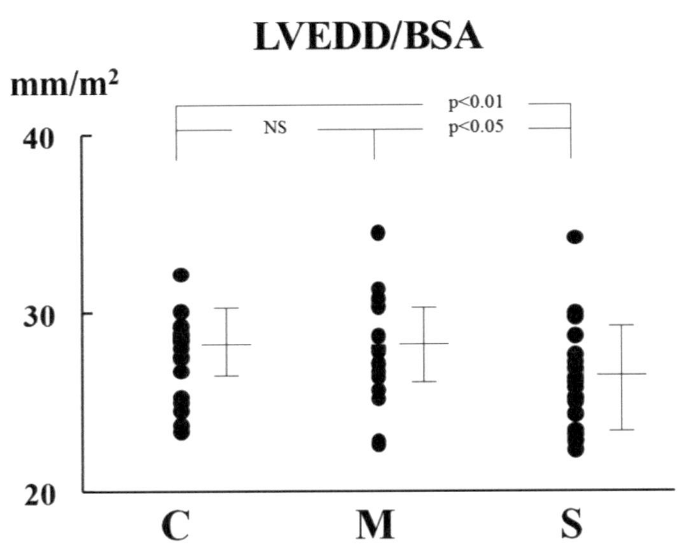

Fig. 4. Comparison of the left ventricular end-diastolic dimension/body surface area (LVEDD/BSA) among the study groups. The mean LVEDD/BSA was significantly lower in S (patients with small heart syndrome and severe symptoms) than in M (patients with small heart syndrome and mild symptoms) and C (control subjects). No significant difference was found between M and C.

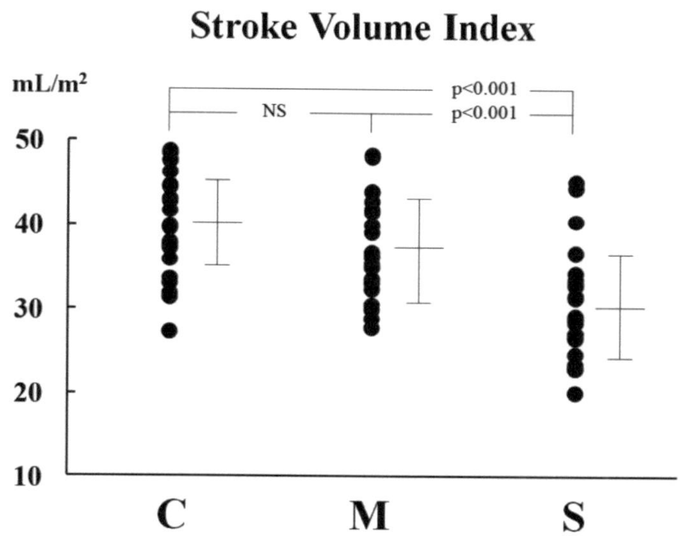

Fig. 5. Comparison of the stroke volume index among the study groups. The mean stroke volume index was significantly lower in S (patients with small heart syndrome and severe symptoms) than in M (patients with small heart syndrome and mild symptoms) and C (control subjects). No significant difference was found between M and C.

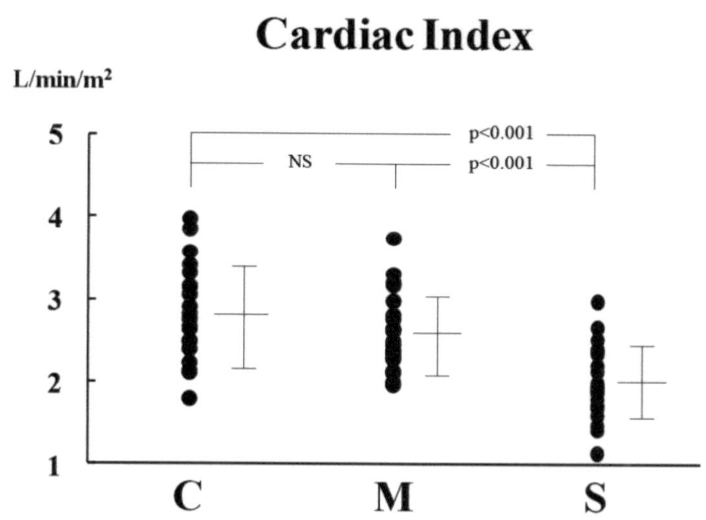

Fig. 6. Comparison of the cardiac index among the study groups. The mean cardiac index was significantly lower in S (patients with small heart syndrome and severe symptoms) than in M (patients with small heart syndrome and mild symptoms) and C (control subjects). No significant difference was found between M and C.

	Control (C)		Small heart syndrome		
			Mild (M)		Severe (S)
		p value		p value	
Number of patients	24		22		25
Sex (male/female)	8/16		7/15		8/17
Age (years)	32±8	NS	30±7	NS	28±6
Body height (cm)	161±9	NS	163±8	NS	163±9
Body weight (kg)	63±17	<0.01	52±10	NS	50±10*
Body mass index (kg/m²)	24±5	<0.001	19±2	NS	18±2†
Body surface area (m²)	1.67±0.24	NS	1.56±0.17	NS	1.53±0.17‡
Cardiothoracic ratio (%)	45±2	<0.001	40±3	NS	38±4†
Heart rate (beats/min)	70±11	NS	71±12	NS	68±11
IVST (mm)	8.8±1.2	NS	8.4±0.9	NS	8.3±1.4
LVPWT (mm)	9.0±1.0	<0.01	8.2±1.1	NS	7.9±1.3*
LVEDD (mm)	46±5	<0.05	43±2	<0.001	39±4†
LVEDD/BSA (mm/m²)	28±2	NS	28±3	<0.05	26±3*
LVESD (mm)	28±3	NS	26±3	NS	25±4†
LVESD/BSA (mm/m²)	17±2	NS	17±2	NS	16±3
LAD (mm)	28±5	NS	25±3	NS	25±4
AoD (mm)	27±4	NS	25±3	NS	25±3
RVD (mm)	15±4	NS	16±3	NS	16±4
Stroke volume (mL)	68±16	<0.001	58±9	<0.001	46±12†
Stroke volume index (mL/m²)	40±6	NS	37±6	<0.001	30±7†
Cardiac output (L/min)	4.7±1.2	<0.05	4.0±0.6	<0.001	3.1±0.8†
Cardiac index (L/min/m²)	2.8±0.6	NS	2.6±0.5	<0.001	2.0±0.4†
Cardiac index <2 L/min/m²	1 (4%)	NS	2 (9%)	<0.01	15 (60%)*
Fractional shortening (%)	39±3	NS	38±5	NS	37±5
Ejection fraction (%)	69±4	NS	69±6	NS	68±6
Mitral valve prolapse	0 (0%)	NS	3 (14%)	NS	4 (16%)

M: patients with small heart syndrome and mild symptoms, S: patients with small heart syndrome and severe symptoms, IVST: interventricular septum thickness, LVPWT: left ventricular posterior wall thickness, LVEDD: left ventricular end-diastolic dimension, LVESD: left ventricular end-systolic dimension, LAD: left atrial dimension, AoD: aortic root diameter, RVD: right ventricular dimension, NS: not significant, *: p<0.01 vs. C, †: p<0.001 vs. C, ‡: p<0.05 vs. C

Table 2. Comparison of the echocardiographic findings among study groups

As shown in Table 2, both the mean body weight and body mass index were significantly lower in both S and M than in C, although the mean body height was not significantly different among the study groups. The mean body surface area was also significantly ($p<0.05$) smaller in S than in C, although the difference was not significant between M and C. The mean CTR (%) values were in the order of S (38±4) < M (40±3) < C (45±2). CTR was significantly ($p<0.001$) lower in S and M than in C, although no significant difference was noted between S and M.

The results of the echocardiographic examination are shown in Table 2 and Figures 3-6. The LV posterior wall (mm) was significantly ($p<0.01$) thinner in S (7.9±1.3) and M (8.2±1.1) than in C (9.0±1.0), although interventricular septum thickness was not significantly different among the groups. The mean LV end-diastolic dimension (LVEDD) (mm) values were in the order of S (39±4) < M (43±2) < C (46±5) (Figure 3). LVEDD was significantly smaller in S ($p<0.001$) and larger in C ($p<0.05$) than in M. The mean LVEDD/body surface area (mm/m^2) was significantly smaller in S (26±3) than in M (28±3, $p<0.05$) and C (28±2, $p<0.01$) (Figure 4). No significant difference was noted in the mean value of LVEDD/body surface area between M and C. In addition, the mean LV end-systolic dimension (LVESD) (mm) values were in the order of S (25±4) < M (26±3) < C (28±3). LVESD was significantly ($p<0.001$) smaller in S than in C. The mean LVESD/body surface area (mm/m^2) was not significantly different among S (16±3), M (17±2) and C (17±2).

Both mean stroke volume and cardiac output values were in the order of S < M < C. Both values were significantly smaller in S and larger in C than in M. The mean stroke volume index (mL/m^2) was significantly ($p<0.001$) smaller in S (30±7) than in M (37±6) and C (40±6) (Figure 5). The mean cardiac index (L/min/m^2) was significantly ($p<0.001$) smaller in S (2.0±0.4) than in M (2.6±0.5) and in C (2.8±0.6) (Figure 6). No significant difference was noted in the mean value of stroke volume index or cardiac index between M and C. The prevalence of low cardiac index (<2 L/min/m^2) was significantly ($p<0.01$) higher in S (60%) than in M (9%) and C (4%). LV ejection fraction (%) was quite comparable among S (68±6), M (69±6) and C (69±4). Mitral valve prolapse was diagnosed in some of the subjects in S (16%) and M (14%).

Thus, we concluded that in patients with a small heart shadow on a chest roentgenogram, a small LV size was generally associated with low cardiac output, which was particularly

Small heart syndrome
postulated by Master in 1944

1) Small heart shadow on chest roentgenogram
2) Hypotension and/or orthostatic dysregulation
3) General malaise, easy fatigability, dizziness, palpitation, dyspnea, chest pain, headedness and cold feet
4) No organic heart disease or systemic disease
5) Thin physiques, asthenia, visceroptosis and wandering kidney
6) Straight back and flat chest
7) Often complicated with mitral valve prolapse syndrome
8) Young female dominant
9) Naïve, delicate and serious character

Fig. 7. Characterization of the patients with small heart syndrome.

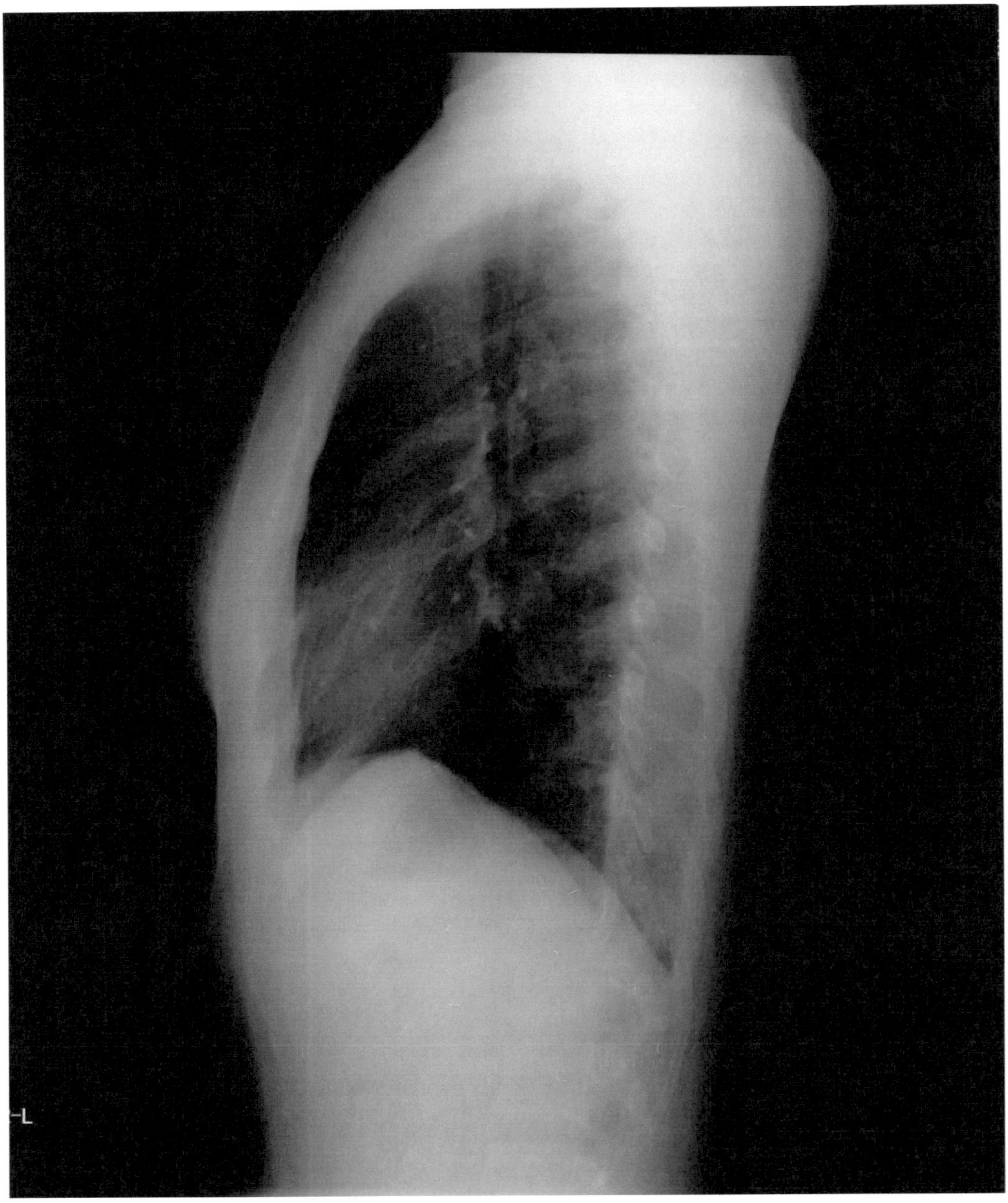

Fig. 8. A typical "straight back" observed in a lateral view chest roentgenogram obtained from a 18-year-old female patient with small heart syndrome.

marked in the patients with severe symptoms and therefore, the pathognomonic significance of a small heart should be recognized as a constitutional factor that predisposes individuals to low output syndrome.[28]

Patients with small heart syndrome are known to have slender structures with low body mass indexes, frequently visceral ptosis with wandering kidney, asthenia, nervousness as well as foot coldness, suggesting physical, autonomic nervous and psychological irritability or lack of relaxation (Figure 7).[11,22,28,29] Thoracic skeletal abnormalities such as shallow chest, straight thoracic spine or loss of the physiologic thoracic kyphosis (Figure 8), and scoliosis are frequently noted in the patients.[11,22,30-32] Mitral valve prolapse[33,34] associated with symptoms such as chest pain, palpitation and dyspnea is a frequent complication of patients with small heart syndrome.[11,22,24,30-32] Many of the small heart subjects appeared to be emotionally sensitive, often delicate and nervous. These conditions may be genetically determined, although several other factors may also be involved in the constitution.[22]

In order to work and perform other duties without excessive exhaustion patients with small heart syndrome need to have enough rest and both physical and emotional relaxation.[11,12] Various triggers including loss of appetite, diarrhea and summer sweating can cause dehydration resulting in preload reduction. It is possible that further reductions in cardiac performance due to preload reduction play an important role in predisposing subjects with small hearts to symptoms including general malaise, fatigue, dizziness, orthostatic dysregulation, dyspnea on effort and palpitations. Autonomic nervous dysfunction with possible accentuated basal parasympathetic tone may be associated with these symptoms through the inhibition of sympathetic activation, which is required to preserve proper cardiac function.[13] Habitual exercise, which can facilitate autonomic nervous adaptation and induce pulmonary and cardiovascular conditioning, may improve the functional work capacity and fatigue by increasing cardiac output. Diarrhea, sweating and loss of appetite as triggering factors for exacerbation should be avoided or treated properly. Constitutional change or conversion is not easy. They may need to take holidays occasionally. And people in their work place and society should understand their specific needs.

2.2 Small heart syndrome as an unrecognized cause of CFS

Recently it has been reported that chest roentgenographic, electrocardiographic and, echocardiographic examinations revealed several distinct findings in CFS patients.[11-13] Specifically, a small heart shadow was often observed on the chest roentgenogram in these patients. In 2008 we first reported that "small heart" with low cardiac output demonstrated by both roentgenographically and echocardiography is prevalent in CFS patients.[11] In this report. small heart syndrome (CTR ≤42%) was significantly more prevalent in the CFS group (n=56) (61%) than in the control group (n=38) (24%) (Table 3). In CFS patients with a small heart (n=34), narrow chest (88%), orthostatic dizziness (44%), foot coldness (41%), pretibial pitting edema (32%), r-kidney palpability (47%), and mitral valve prorapse (29%) were all significantly more prevalent than in the control group, and also in the CFS patients without small heart syndrome (Table 4). Echocardiographic examination demonstrated significantly smaller values of both LV end-diastolic and end-systolic dimensions, and stroke volume and cardiac indexes in CFS with a small heart as compared with control subjects with a normal heart size (42%< CTR <50%) (Table 5). Thus, a considerable number of CFS patients have a small heart and cardiac performance is actually impaired with low cardiac output due to a small LV chamber size and poor cardiac function with low stroke volume and cardiac indexes in many of CFS patients.[11] In addition, both the reduced cardiac size and performance during the exacerbation phase was improved during the remission phase in

CFS patients with "small heart", suggesting that small heart syndrome with impaired cardiac function may play an important role in the genesis of CFS (Table 6).[12] Also cardiothoracic ratios increased significantly during the remission phase as compared with exacerbation phase (Table 6).[12] Reduced LV ejection fraction was not observed in any patients, suggesting no myocardial systolic dysfunction. Many CFS patients have low cardiac output and the resulting low flow circulatory state may make it difficult for patients to meet the demands of everyday activity, and it may also lead to fatigue and other conditions. Small heart syndrome may contribute to the development of CFS as a constitutional factor predisposing to fatigue, and may be included in the genesis of CFS.

	Control	CFS	p
n	38	56	
Gender (male/female)	19/19	26/30	NS
Age (year)	36±8	33±8	NS
Body mass index	22±3	21±5	NS
CTR (%)			
≤42	9 (24%)	34 (61%)	p<0.01
≤40	6 (16%)	25 (45%)	p<0.01
Narrow chest	7 (18%)	33 (59%)	p<0.01

CFS: Chronic fatigue syndrome; CTR: cardiothoracic ratio; NS: not significant

Table 3. Comparison of chest roentgenographic and physical examination findings in study patients

	Control	CFS Small heart (-)	CFS Small heart (+)	p value
n	38	22	34	
Male/female	19/19	13/9	13/21	
Age (year)	36±8	34±8	31±8	<0.05*
Body mass index	22±3	25±6	19±3	<0.001*
Narrow chest	7 (18%)	4 (18%)	30 (88%)	<0.01*
Orthostatic dizziness	5 (13%)	3 (14%)	15 (44%)	<0.05*
Foot coldness	4 (11%)	2 (9%)	14 (41%)	<0.05*
Pretibial pitting edema	3 (8%)	1 (5%)	11 (32%)	<0.05*
r-kidney palpability	4 (11%)	1(5%)	1 (47%)	<0.01*
Mitral valve prolapse	3 (8%)	0 (0%)	10 (29%)	<0.05*

*: vs. Control and Small heart (-)
CFS: Chronic fatigue syndrome

Table 4. Comparison of physical examination findings in control and CFS, with and without a small heart

Indeed, CFS patients had a variety of possible cardiovascular complaints, including chest pain, palpitation, dyspnea or shortness of breath, coldness of feet, dizziness and fainting, although all of these symptoms are not necessarily attributable to cardiovascular dysfunction.[13] Frequently noted physical examination findings such as epigastric splash sound, right kidney palpability, cold feet and pretibial pitting edema, may be related to visceral ptosis with slender build, and peripheral circulatory impairment.[13] Weakness, rapid heartbeat and orthostatic dizziness may be related to hypotension and orthostatic dysregulation. Auscultatory findings including a late systolic murmur and a mid-systolic click suggested typical mitral valve prolapse in some of the patients. In addition, electrocardiograms showed severe sinus arrhythmia and vertical or right axis deviation in a considerable number of the patients, suggesting parasympathetic predominance and vertical heart position.[13] Following our reports Hurwitz et al.[14] reported that severe CFS patients had lower cardiac output associated with lower cardiac volume indicated echocardiographically and lower total blood volume, plasma volume and red blood cell volume indicated by dual tag blood volume assessments as compared with controls, suggesting a co-morbid hypovolemic condition.

	Control 50%>CTR>42%	CFS with small heart CTR≤42%	p value
n	30	34	
Male/female	11/19	13/21	NS
Age (y)	34±13	31±8	0.219
Body height (cm)	163±7	164±10	0.451
Body weight (kg)	60±16	53±11	0.040*
Body surface area (m^2)	1.6±0.2	1.6±0.2	0.146
Heart rate (beats/min)	69±12	72±13	0.363
IVS (mm)	9±1	9±1	0.574
PW (mm)	9±1	8±1	0.709
LVEDD (mm)	45±4	41±5	0.002*
LVESD (mm)	28±3	25±5	0.038*
LAD (mm)	27±5	25±4	0.229
AoD (mm)	27±5	26±4	0.261
RAD (mm)	15±3	16±4	0.361
Stroke volume (ml)	65±14	52±14	0.001*
Stroke volume index (ml/m^2)	39±7	33±8	0.001*
Cardiac output (l/min)	4.4±1.2	3.7±1.0	0.005*
Cardiac index (l/min/m^2)	2.7±0.6	2.3±0.6	0.012*
Fractional shortening (%)	39±4	37±4	0.188
Ejection fraction (%)	69±4	68±5	0.313

*: significant
IVS: interventrricular septum thickness; PW: LV posterior wall thickness; EDD: end-diastolic dimension; ESD: end-systolic dimension; LAD: left atrial dimension; AoD: aortic root diameter; RVD; right ventricular dimension
CFS: chronic fatigue syndrome

Table 5. Comparison of echocardiographic findings in control with a normal heart size and CFS with a small heart

	Exacerbatioin	Remission	p value
Heart rate (beats/min)	71±9	63±6	0.014*
LVEDD (mm)	38±4	43±3	<0.001*
LVESD (mm)	24±2	27±2	0.015*
Stroke volume (ml)	41±10	56±11	<0.001*
Stroke volume index (ml/m²)	28±7	39±6	<0.001*
Cardiac output (l/min)	2.8±0.6	3.6±0.9	0.017*
Cardiac index (l/min/ m²)	2.0±0.4	2.5±0.5	0.014*
Ejection Fraction (%)	66±3	68±6	0.443
CTR (%)	38±2	40±2	<0.001*

LV: left ventricular; EDD: end-diastolic dimension; ESD: end-systolic dimension; CTR: cardiothoracic ratio

*: statistically significant

Table 6. Comparison of echocardiographic findings of 10 CFS patients with a small heart between the exacerbation and remission phases

3. Orthostatic Intolerance (OI)

Patients with orthostatic intolerance have been clinically recognized.[35-37] The patients predictably develop symptoms of disabling fatigue, dizziness, diminished concentration, tremulousness, and nausea while standing (Table 7). Simple activities such as eating, showering, or low intensity exercise may profoundly exacerbate these symptoms. Reduced cerebral blood flow with impaired cerebral oxygenation during an upright posture is considered as major mechanism for orthostatic intolerance,[17,38] although compensatory sympathetic activation also seems to play an important role in the development of the

Symptoms While Standing in Patients with Orthostatic Intolerance
Disabling fatigue
General malaise
Diminished concentration
Dizziness
Fainting
Pallolr
Weakness
Tremulousness
Sweating
Light headedness
Visual disturbance
Palpitations
Dyspnea
Nausea
Nervousness

Table 7. Symptoms while standing in patients with orthostatic intolerance

various symptoms in cases it is exaggerated.[36-41] Assuming an upright posture causes translocation of approximately 800 ml of blood from the intrathoracic venous compartment to veins of the buttocks, pelvis and legs.[42] The normal compensatory cardiovascular response to this orthostatic stress is a neurogenically mediated increase in heart rate and in systemic vascular resistance.[42] Not all vascular beds contribute equally to the reflex increase in vascular resistance.[42] Splanchnic vasoconstriction accounts for one third, and skin and muscle vasoconstriction, approximately 40% of the increased vascular resistance during normal levels orthostatic stress.[42] Symptoms of orthostatic intolerance develop as these reflexes approach the limit of compensation.

3.1 Similarities and overlaps between CFS and OI

Many of the primary symptoms of orthostatic intolerance are often seen in patients with disabling CFS.[17,42,43] Both CFS and orthostatic intolerance affects many young people, predominantly women. Many symptoms of OI appear to be related to reduced cerebral blood flow. Symptoms are associated with inadequate systemic venous return to the right heart or thoracic hypovolemia,[35,36] although precise mechanisms remain to be clarified. Also excessive lower body venous pooling with delayed orthostatic hypotension, by reducing cerebral perfusion, has been suggested to be involved in the orthostatic component of fatigue in CFS patients.[44]

3.2 Pathopysiology of OI

Potential pathophysiological mechanisms in chronic orthostatic intolerance include a β-adrenergic hypersensitivity,[45] decreased plasma volume,[46] an inappropriate venous pooling,[44] and possible dysautonomia.[36-41,47] Several disorders including delayed orthostatic hypotension,[17] neurally mediated hypotension[48] and postural orthostatic tachycardia syndrome[35-38] underlies or promotes orthostatic intolerance. Delayed orthostatic hypotension can be caused by excessive gravitational venous pooling.[17,44] Impaired vasoconstrictor function with relative bradycardia is often seen in neurally mediated hypotension.[48] In 1995 Rowe et al.[48] described the cases with an overlap in the symptoms of CFS and neurally mediated hypotension, suggesting that neurally mediated hypotension should be considered as a treatable cause of CFS. Exaggerated tachycardia and vasoconstriction without hypotension of postural orthostatic tachycardia syndrome (POTS) during standing can cause orthostatic intolerance,[35-38] although pathophysiology of POTS remains unclear. In 1982 Rosen and Cryer were the first to describe a woman with a 7-year history of disabling postural tachycardia and palpitations in association with an idiopathic reduction in plasma volume.[35] In 1993 Schondorf and Low[36] reviewed the patients who exhibited exaggerated tachycardia at rest or during head-up tilt and named "idiopathic postural orthostatic tachycardia syndrome" which may be a manifestation of a mild form of acute autonomic neuropathy. Studies suggest that POTS is accompanied with a range of autonomic nervous system abnormalities including vagal withdrawal and enhanced sympathetic modulation, associated with findings consistent with pooling in the lower limbs.[36-41,44,47] Also studies in adolescents suggest that POTS physiology underlies OI in the majority of CFS patients.[41-44] POTS is a frequent finding in patients with CFS.[41-44] Clinical evaluation of CFS patients should include response to standing. POTS may be an under-recognized condition in CFS as Hoad et al.[49] recently suggested.

3.3 OI and small heart

Recently it has been reported that patients with postural orthostatic tachycardia, which is often noted in patients with chronic orthostatic intolerance, had a smaller heart coupled with reduced blood volume compared with healthy controls.[50] By using a cardiac magnetic resonance imaging technique, Fu et al.[50] assessed precisely the heart size and mass in POTS patients and found that cardiac size and mass and blood volume were much smaller in the patients compared with healthy sedentary controls. The marked orthostatic tachycardia in these patients seemed to be a physiologic compensatory response to a smaller stroke volume and exercise training improved this syndrome in most patients.[50] Fu et al.[50] offered POTS a new name based on its underlying pathophysiology, the "Grinch syndrome", because in this famous children's book by Dr Seuss, the main character had a heart that was "two sizes too small". In their assessment of both sympathetic baroreflex sensitivity and cardiovagal baroreflex sensitivity, the function of autonomic nervous system was intact in the patients,[50] although other researchers have postulated autonomic nervous dysfunction with exaggerated sympathetic nervous activation over compensatory levels during standing as a major mechanism for the symptoms.[35,36,40,41,47]

Although some dysautonomia cause orthostatic instability accompanied with abnormal changes in heart rate and blood pressure, whether disorders of the autonomic nervous system is responsible for OI and also OI in CFS patients is controversial.[38,39,43,44,50] Recently, Jones et al.[51] reported that orthostatic instability was similar in persons with CFS and nonfatigued control subjects recruited from the general Wichita population. Interestingly persons with higher serum osmolarity levels had significantly higher abnormal tilt rates than those with lower serum osmolarity levels, suggesting that delayed responses to head-up tilt tests may reflect hydration status.[51] Reappraisal of primary dysautomia as a factor in the pathogenesis of CFS and also OI may be needed. In the meanwhile Ewan et al.[52] reported that use of the sinus node blocker ivabradine led to dramatic improvements in subjective and objective symptomatology in line with a reduction in heart rate on standing in a 21 year-old female patient with POTS. Use of this medication appears to not only improve tachycardia but also symptomatology, including fatigue, suggesting that tachycardia is not only unnecessary for maintaining cerebral perfusion while standing as a compensatory mechanism but also triggers many symptoms possibly through disturbances in autonomic nervous system.

3.4 Pronounced small heart in CFS with OI

We aimed to test a hypothesis that small heart is associated with OI in patients with CFS. Among the 46 study CFS patients, 26 (57%) were classified as CFSOI according to the presence of OI. In addition, 11 OI patients and 27 age- and sex-matched control subjects (Controls) were studied. Left ventricular (LV) dimensions and function were determined echocardiographically. As shown in Table 8 and Figures 9-11, the mean values of cardiothoracic ratio, systemic systolic and diastolic pressures, LV end-diastolic dimensions, LV end-systolic dimensions, stroke volume indexes, cardiac indexes and LV mass indexes were all significantly smaller in CFSOI and OI than in Controls. A smaller LV end-diastolic dimension (< 40 mm) was significantly more prevalently noted in CFSOI (54%) and OI (45%) than in Controls (4%). A lower cardiac index (< 2 l/min/mm^2) was more prevalent in CFSOI (65%) than in OI (27%) and Controls (11%). The mean values of both LV fractional shortening and ejection fraction were comparable among the groups (Table 8). In conclusion, a small size of

LV with low cardiac output was noted in OI and marked in CFSOI. A small heart appears to be related to the genesis of OI and CFS via both cerebral and systemic hypoperfusion. CFSOI seems to constitute a well-defined and predominant subgroup of CFS.

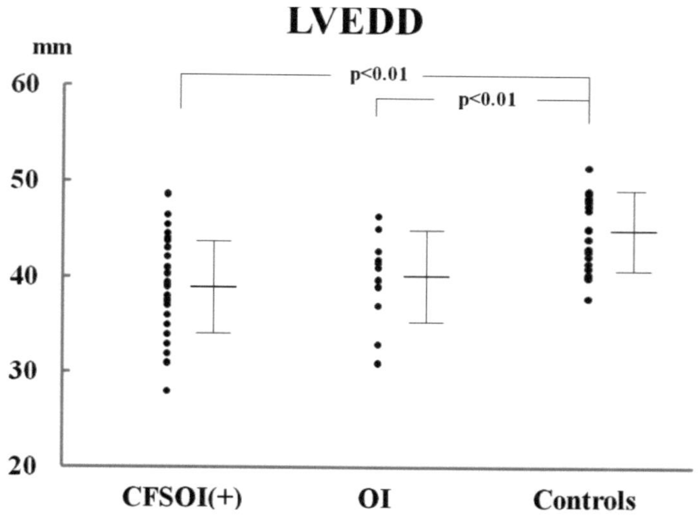

CFSOI: patients with chronic fatigue syndrome and orthostatic intolerance
OI: patients with orthostatic intolerance but without chronic fatigue syndrome
Controls: healthy control subjects

Fig. 9. Comparison of the left ventricular end-diastolic dimensions (LVEDD) among the study groups.

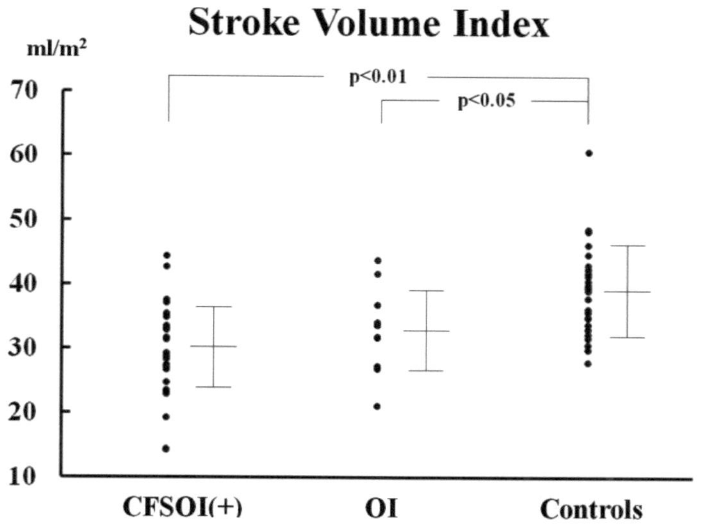

CFSOI: patients with chronic fatigue syndrome and orthostatic intolerance
OI: patients with orthostatic intolerance but without chronic fatigue syndrome
Controls: healthy control subjects

Fig. 10. Comparison of the stroke volume indexes among the study groups.

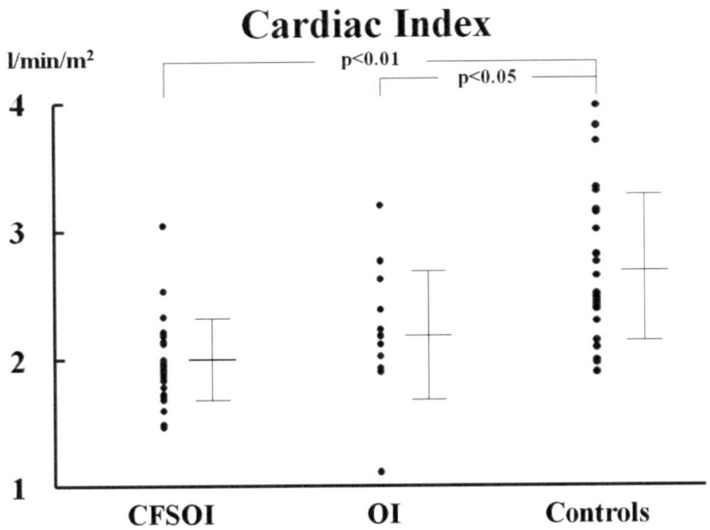

CFSOI: patients with chronic fatigue syndrome and orthostatic intolerance
OI: patients with orthostatic intolerance but without chronic fatigue syndrome
Controls: healthy control subjects

Fig. 11. Comparison of the cardiac indexes among the study groups.

Elucidation of the pathophysiology of CFS and OI may lead to better therapeutic strategies. Recently, xenon-computed tomography blood flow studies demonstrated that CFS patients have global cerebral hypoperfusion with reduced absolute cortical blood flow in broad areas, especially in bilateral middle cerebral artery territories, compared with healthy controls.[53] Impaired cerebral oxygenation due to reduced cerebral hemodynamics in young CFS with OI during an active standing test was suggested from the findings of continuous measurement of cerebral oxygenated hemoglobin using near-infrared spectroscopy.[54] In the present study, low systolic and diastolic blood pressures were noted in OI patients with and without CFS compared with those in control subjects. Newton et al.[55] have consolidated the evidence using 24-hour ambulatory blood pressure monitoring that lower blood pressure occurs in CFS patients and lower nighttime blood pressure seems to be a significant problem that may lead to the enhanced diurnal variation. The putative mechanism by which OI and CFS are triggered or caused in patients with a small heart is shown in Figure 12.

	CFSOI	OI	Controls
Number of patients	26	11	27
Male/Female	7/19	2/9	10/17
Age (years)	28±8	31±7	32±7
Cardiothoracic ratio (%)	38±5†	42±3‡	44±4
Heart rate (beats/min)	69±15	68±11	70±12
Systolic blood pressure (mmHg)	109±11*	112±14†	121±11
Diastolic blood pressure (mmHg)	66±12*	68±13†	75±12
IVS (mm)	8±1	8±1	9±1
PW (mm)	8±1	8±1	9±1
LVEDD (mm)	39±5*	40±5*	45±4
<40	14 (54%)*	5 (45%)*	1 (4%)
LVESD (mm)	25±5*	24±5*	27±2
LAD (mm)	25±5	24±4	27±4
AoD (mm)	26±4	25±3	27±5
RVD (mm)	15±4	15±2	15±3
Stroke volume (ml)	45±13*	49±11*	63±13
Stroke volume index (ml/m^2)	30±7*	33±7†	39±7
Cardiac output (l/min)	3.0±0.7*	3.3±1.0*	4.4±1.0
Cardiac index (l/min/m^2)	2.0±0.3*†	2.2±0.5†	2.7±0.6
< 2	17 (65%)*	3 (27%)	3 (11%)
Fractional shortening (%)	37±4	40±7	39±3
LV Ejection fraction (%)	67±5	71±8	69±4
LV mass index (g/m^2)	62±16†	64±13‡	77±16

IVS: interventricular septum thickness; PW: left ventricular (LV) posterior wall thickness; LVEDD: LV end-diastolic dimension; LVESD: LV end-systolic dimension; LAD: left atrial dimension; AoD: aortic root diameter; RVD: right ventricular dimension
*: p <0.01 vs. Controls †: p <0.05 vs. Controls
Comparisons of values between the study groups were performed with ANOVA followed by Student's unpaired t-test. Proportional data were analyzed by the chi-square test, with Yates' correction.

Table 8. Comparative echocardiographic data among the study groups

Reasonable potentiation of cerebrovascular flow without exaggerated activation or perturbation of autonomic nervous system may be needed for effective treatment. However, administration of nonselective vasoconstrictive agents may cause a simple reduction of cerebral blood flow via elevation of cerebrovascular resistance, although intravenous infusion of phenylephrine, a sympathetic nerve α_1 stimulator, has been reported to improve OI, as a result of producing significant peripheral vasoconstriction and venoconstriction in some OI patients.[56] Volume repletion by increasing sodium intake or by treatment with fludrocortisones may theoretically improve OI and also symptoms of CFS by replenishing intravascular volume.[17,35,38,42,46] Military anti-shock trousers as well as elastic stockings which compress lower extremities may also be effective via potentiation of venous return, resulting in increased cardiac output.[44] Although CFS patients are limited by the discomfort of an increased perception of exertion, there are some data to support the notion that an appropriately designed exercise program is beneficial.[50,57-59] Various triggers including loss of appetite, diarrhea and sweating can cause dehydration accompanied by preload reduction, leading to further decreases in stroke volume and cardiac output, thereby impairing both systemic and cerebral circulation and exacerbating symptoms, and therefore should be avoided or treated appropriately.

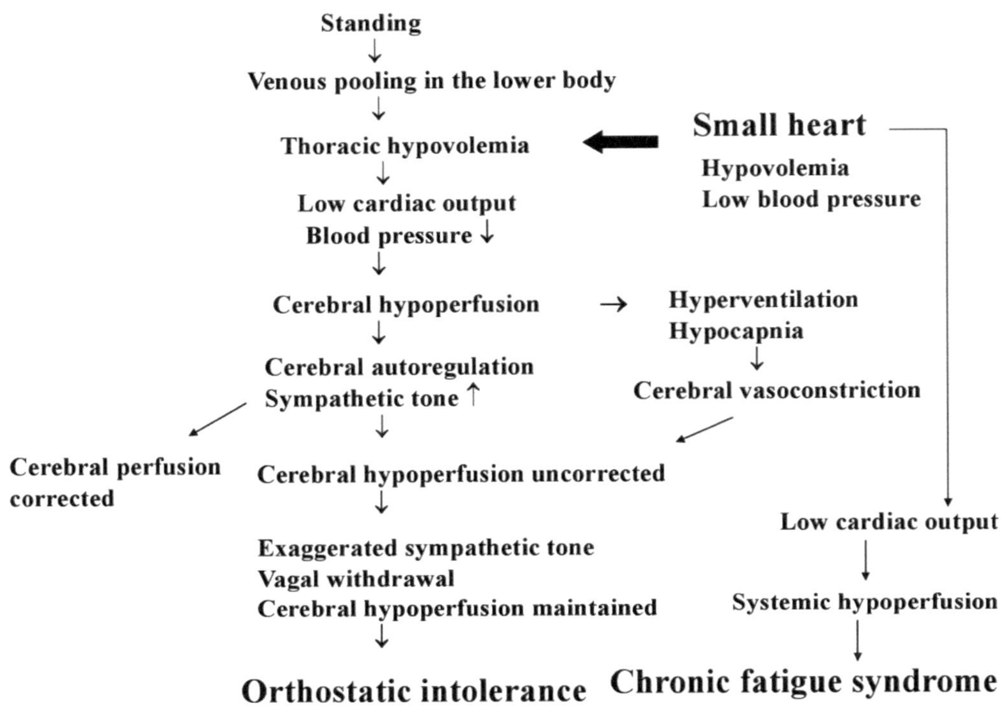

Fig. 12. The putative mechanism by which orthostatic intolerance and chronic fatigue syndrome are triggered in patients with a small heart.

4. Conclusions

Cardiac dysfunction with low cardiac output due to a small LV chamber may contribute to the development of chronic fatigue as a constitutional factor in a considerable number of CFS patients and its degree appears to be more pronounced in CFS patients with OI.[60] CFS with OI seems to constitute a well-defined and predominant subgroup of CFS. Small heart with reduced cardiac performance due to decreased preload may be an important target for the treatment of CFS.

5. References

[1] Holmes GP, Kaplan JE, Gantz NM, Komaroff AL, Schonberger LB, Straus SE, Jones JF, Dibois RE, Cunningham-Rundles C, Pahwa S, Tosato G, Zegans LS, Purtilo DT, Brown N, Schooley RT, Brus I. Chronic fatigue syndrome: A working case definition. Ann Int Med 1988;108:387-389.

[2] Shafran SD. The chronic fatigue syndrome. Am J Med 1991; 90: 730-739.
[3] Fukuda K, Straus SE, Hickle I, Sharpe Mc, Dobbins JG, Komaroff A, International Chronic Fatigue Syndrome Study Group. The chronic fatigue syndrome: A comprehensive approach to its definition and study. Ann Int Med 1994; 121: 953-959.
[4] Afari N, Buchwald D. Chronic fatigue syndrome: A review. Am J Psychiatry 2003; 160: 221-236.
[5] Klonoff DC. Chronic fatigue syndrome. Clin Inf Dis 1992; 15: 812-823.
[6] Reeves WC, Wagnor D, Nisenbaum R, Jones JF, Gurbaxani B, Solomon L, Papanicolaou DA, Unger ER, Vernon SD, Heim C. Chronic fatigue syndrome—A clinically empirical approach to its definition and study. BMC Medicine 2005; 3: 19-27.
[7] Miwa K, Fujita M. Increased oxidative stress suggested by low serum vitamin E concentrations in patients with chronic fatigue syndrome. Int J Cardiol 2009; 136: 238-239.
[8] Miwa K, Fujita M. Fluctuation of serum vitamin E (α-tocopherol) concentrations during exacerbation and remission phases in patients with chronic fatigue syndrome. Heart Vessels 2010; 25: 319-323.
[9] Montague TJ, Marrie TJ, Klassen GA, Bewick DJ, Horacek BM. Cardiac function at rest and with exercise in the chronic fatigue syndrome Chest 1989; 95: 779-784.
[10] Peckerman A, Lamanca JJ, Dahl KA, Chemitiganti R, Qureishi B, Natelson BH. Abnormal impedance cardiography predicts symptom severity in chronic fatigue syndrome. Am J Med Sci 2003; 326: 55-60.
[11] Miwa K, Fujita M. "Small heart syndrome" in patients with chronic fatigue syndrome. Clin Cardiol 2008; 31: 328-333.
[12] Miwa K, Fujita M. Cardiac function fluctuates during exacerbation and remission in young adults with chronic fatigue syndrome and "small heart". J Cardiol 2009; 54: 29-35.
[13] Miwa K, Fujita M. Cardiovascular dysfunction with low cardiac output due to small heart in patients with chronic fatigue syndrome. Inter Med 2009; 48: 1849-1854.
[14] Hurwitz BE, Coryell VT, Parker M, Martin P, LaPerriere A, Kilmas NG, Sfakianakis GN, Bilsker MS. Chronic fatigue syndrome: illness severity, sedentary lifestyle, blood volume and evidence of diminished cardiac function. Clin Sci 2010; 118:125-135.
[15] Cordero DL, Sisto SA, Tapp WN, Lamanca JJ, Pareja JG, Natelson BH. Decreased vagal power during treadmill walking in patients with chronic fatigue syndrome. Clin Auton Res 1996; 6: 329-333.
[16] Yataco A, Talo H, Rowe P, Kass DA, Berger RD, Calkins H. Comparison of heart rate variability in patients with chronic fatigue syndrome and controls. Clin Auton Res 1997; 7: 293-297.
[17] Streeten DHP, Thomas D, Bell DS. The roles of orthostatic hypotension, orthostatic tachycardia, and subnormal erythrocyte volume in the pathogenesis of the chronic fatigue syndrome. Am J Med Sci 2000; 320: 1-8.
[18] Freeman R, Lirofonis V, Farquhar WB, Risk M. Limb venous compliance in patients with idiopathic orthostatic intolerance and postural tachycardia. J Appl Physiol 2002; 93: 636-644.

[19] Bakheit AM, Behan PO, Watson WS, Morton JJ. Abnormal arginine-vasopression secretion and water metabolism in patients with postviral fatigue syndrome. Acta Neurol Scand 1993; 87: 234-238.
[20] Ottenweller JE, Sisto SA, McCarty RC, Natelson BH. Hormonal responses to exercise to chronic fatigue syndrome. Neuropsychobiology 2001; 43: 34-41.
[21] Laennec RTH: Traité de L'auscultation Mdiate et des Maladies des Poumons et du Coeur. (Eds. Chaude JS), pp 496-497, JS Chaude, Paris, 1826.
[22] Master AM. Neurocirculatory asthenia due to small heart. Med Clin North Am 1944; 28: 577-588.
[23] DaCosta JM. An irritable heart; a clinical study of a form of functional cardiac disorder and its consequences. Am J Med Sci 1871; 121: 17-53.
[24] Wooley CF. Where are the Diseases of Yesteryear? DaCosta's syndrome, soldiers heart, the effort syndrome, neurocirculatory asthenia—And the mitral valve prolapse syndrome. Circulation 1976; 53: 749-751.
[25] Takahashi T, Sakamoto T, Hada Y, Amano K, Yamaguchi T, Takikawa R, Hasegawa I, Takahashi H, Sugimoto T. Echocardiographic features of small heart. J Cardiol 1985; 15: 867-875. (in Japanese with English abstract)
[26] Schiller NB, Shah PM, Crawford M, DeMaria A, Devereux R, Feigenbaum H, Gutgeseaell H, Reichek N, Sahn D, Schnittinger I, Silverman N, Tajik J, the American Society of Echocardiography, Committee on Standards, Subcommittee on Quantification of Two-Dimensional Echocardiograms. Recommendations for the quantification of the left ventricle by two-dimensional echocardiography. J Am Soc Echocardiogr 1989; 2: 358-367.
[27] Teichholz LE, Kreulen T, Herman MV, Gorlin R. Problems in echocardiographic volume determinations: Echocardiographic-angiographic correlations in the presence or absence of asynergy. Am J Cardiol 1976 ; 37:7-11.
[28] Miwa K, Fujita M. Is small heart syndrome a "heart" disease or low output syndrome? Int J Cardiol 2011; 146 : 95-96.
[29] Abe T. The small heart syndrome. Asian Med J 1990; 33: 295-302.
[30] Tempo CPB, Ronan Jr JA, deLeon Jr AC, Twigg HL. Radiographic appearance of the thorax in systolic click-late systolic murmur syndrome. Am J Cardiol 1975; 36: 27-31.
[31] Salomon J, Shah PM, Heinle RA. Thoracic skeletal abnormalities in idiopathic mitral valve prolapse. Am J Cardiol 1975; 36: 32-36.
[32] Udoshi MB, Shah A, Fisher VJ, Dolgin M. Incidence of mitral valve prolapse in subjects with thoracic skeletal abnormalities - A prospective study. Am Heart J 1979; 97: 303-311.
[33] Gilbert BW, Schatz RA, Van Ramm OT, Behar VS, Kisslo JA. Mitral valve prolapse: Two-dimensional echocardiographic and angiographic correlation. Circulation 1976; 54: 716-723.
[34] Yoshikawa J, Kato H, Yanagihara K, Okumachi F, Takagi Y, Yoshida K, Asaka Y, Inanami H. Criteria for the diagnosis of prolapsed mitral valve using phonocardiography and echocardiography. J Cardiography 1982; 12: 773-777. (in Japanese with English abstract)

[35] Rosen S, Cryer PE. Postural tachycardia syndrome. Reversal of sympathetic hyperreponsiveness and clinical improvement during sodium loading. Am J Med 1982; 72: 847-850.
[36] Schondorf R, Low PA. Idiopathic postural orthostatic tachycardia syndrome: An attenuated form of acute pandysautonomia? Neurology 1993; 43:132-137.
[37] Robertson D. The epidemic of orthostatic tachycardia and orthostatic intolerance. Am J Med Sci 1999; 317:75-77.
[38] Stewart J. Chronic orthostatic intolerance and the postural tachycardia syndrome (POTS). J Pediatr 2004; 145: 725-730.
[39] Furlan R, Jacob G, Snell M, Robertson D, Porta A, Harris P, Mosqueda-Garcia R. Chronic orthostatic intolerance: a disorder with discordant cardiac and vascular sympathetic control. Circulation 1998; 98: 2154-2159.
[40] Stewart J. Pooling in chronic orthostatic intolerance. Arterial vasoconstrictive but not venous compliance defects. Circulation 2002; 105: 2274-2281.
[41] Stewart J. Autonomic nervous system dysfunction in adolescents with postural orthostatic tachycardia syndrome and chronic fatigue syndrome is characterized by attenuated vagal baroreflex and potentiated sympathetic vasomotion. Pediatric Res 2000; 48: 218-226
[42] Schondorf R, Freeman R. The importance of orthostatic intolerance in the chronic fatigue syndrome. Am J Med Sci 1999; 317: 117-123.
[43] Schondorf R, Benoit J, Wein T, Phaneuf D. Orthostatic intolerance in the chronic fatigue syndrome. J Auton Nerv Syst 1999; 75: 192-201.
[44] Streeten DHP. Role of impaired lower-limb venous innervations in the pathogenesis of the chronic fatigue syndrome. Am J Med Sci 2001; 321: 163-167.
[45] Frohlich ED, Tarazi RC, Dustan HP. Hyperdynamic beta-adrenergic circulatory state. Arch Intern Med 1969; 123: 1-7.
[46] Fouad FM, Tadena-Thome L, Bravo EL, Tarazi RC. Idiopathic hypovolemia. Ann Int Med 1986; 104: 298-303.
[47] Jacobs G, Costa F, Shannon JR, Robertson RM, Wathen M, Stein M, Biaggioni I, Ertl A, Black B, Robertson D. The neuropathic postural tachycardia syndrome. N Engl J Med 2000; 343: 1008-1014.
[48] Rowe PC, Bou-Holaigah I, Kan JS, Calkins H. Is neutrally mediated hypotension an unrecognised cause of chronic fatigue? Lancet 1995; 345: 623-624.
[49] Hoad A Spickett G, Elliot J, Newton J. Postural orthostatic tachycardia syndrome is an under-recognized condition in chronic fatigue syndrome. Q J Med 2008; 101: 961-965.
[50] Fu Q, VanGundy TB, Galbreath M, Shibata S, Jain M, Hastings JL, Bhella PS, Levine BD. Cardiac origins of the postural orthostatic tachycardia syndrome. J Am Coll Cardiol 2010; 55:2858-68.
[51] Jones JF, Nicholson A, Nisenbaum R, Papanicolaou DA, Solomon L, Boneva R, Heim C, Reeves WC. Orthostatic instability in a population-based study of chronic fatigue syndrome. Am J Med 2005; 118: 1415.e19-e28.
[52] Ewan V, Norton M, Newton JL. Symptom improvement in postural orthostatic tachycardia syndrome with the sinus node blocker ivabradine. Europace 2007; 9: 1202.

[53] Yoshiuchi K, Farkas J, Natelson B. Patients with chronic fatigue syndrome have reduced absolute cortical blood flow. Clin Physiol Funct Imaging 2006; 26: 83-86.

[54] Tanaka H, Matsushima R, Tamai H, Kajimoto Y. Impaired postural cerebral hemodynamics in young patients with chronic fatigue with and without orthostatic intolerance. J Pediatr 2002; 140:412-417.

[55] Newton JL, Sheth A, Shin J, Pairman J, Wilton K, Burt JA, Jones DE. Lower ambulatory blood pressure in chronic fatigue syndrome. Psychosomatic Medicine 2009; 71: 361-365.

[56] Stewart J, Munoz J, Weldon A. Clinical and physiological effects of an acute α-1 adrenergic and β-1 adrenergic antagonist in chronic orthostatic intolerance. Circulation 2002; 106: 2946-2954.

[57] Wilson A, Hickie I, Lloyd A, Wakefield D. The treatment of chronic fatigue syndrome: science and speculation. Am J Med 1994; 96:544-550.

[58] Fulcher KY, White PD. Randomised controlled trial of graded exercise in patients with the chronic fatigue syndrome. Br Med J 1997; 314:1647-1657.

[59] Wearden AJ, Morris RK, Mullis R, Strickland PL, Pearson DJ, Appleby L, Campbell IT, Morris JA. Randomised, double-blind, placebo-controlled treatment trial of fluoxetine and graded exercise for chronic fatigue syndrome. Br J Psychiatry 1998; 172: 485-490.

[60] Miwa K, Fujita M. Small heart with low cardiac output for orthostatic intolerance in patients with chronic fatigue syndrome. Clin Cardiol in press. DOI: 10.1002/clc.20962©2011 Wiley Pediodicals, Inc.